CLINICAL VETERINARY MEDICINE -II

Practical Manual Series - 3

Clinical Veterinary Medicine-II

By

Dr. Neelesh Sharma

(Assistant Professor)

Dr. S.R. Upadhyay

(Assistant Professor)

Division of Veterinary Clinical Medicine & Jurisprudence
Faculty of Veterinary Sciences & Animal Husbandry
Sher-e-Kashmir University of Agricultural Sciences & Technology
R.S. Pura, Jammu - 181 102 (J&K), India

2009

New India Publishing Agency

Pitam Pura, New Delhi- 110 088

Published by
Sumit Pal Jain *for*

New India Publishing Agency

101, Vikas Surya Plaza, CU Block, L.S.C. Mkt.,
Pitam Pura, New Delhi- 110 088, (India)
Phone: 011-27341717, Fax: 011-27341616
E-mail: newindiapublishingagency@gmail.com
Web: www.bookfactoryindia.com

ISBN : 978-81-90851-25-1

Typeset at: Typographiya # 9811482328
Printed at: Jai Bharat Printing Press, Delhi

PREFACE

The need of a simple manual explaining the basic principles and procedures to cater the requirements of students is always desirable. Keeping this in view the practical manual in "Clinical Veterinary Medicine", for course no. VCM-512 has been prepared strictly in accordance with the syllabi prescribed for the subject by the Veterinary Council of India. Veterinary Council of India (Minimum standards of Veterinary Education Degree Course- B.V. Sc. & A.H.) Regulations, 1993, have provided necessary curriculum and syllabus for the degree course of B.V. Sc. & A.H.

It is hoped that this manual will help the under graduate students to learn the subject in an interactive and easy manner. It will also aid the teachers to impart instructions in Clinical Veterinary Medicine effectively.

12, March, 2009
Jammu

Dr. Neelash Sharma
Dr. S.R. Upadhyay

INTRODUCTION

Metabolic diseases are the most commonly recognized diseases at dairy farms. While the pathogenesis is well known, metabolic disorders continue to occur. Amongst domestic farm animals, the metabolic diseases have great importance in dairy cows production because the producing dairy cow verges always on abnormal homeostasis. The breeding and feeding of dairy cattle for high milk yield are etiologically related to the metabolic diseases so they are common in these animals. Evidence suggests that metabolic disease affects host defense, and therefore, impacts the common infectious diseases of dairy cows. Metabolic diseases are those associated with the chemical processes necessary for maintenance of life. In cattle, metabolic diseases include errors in electrolyte / mineral metabolism, of which parturient hypocalcemia (milk fever) is most common, or errors associated with energy metabolism, including ketosis and displaced abomasum. Metabolic diseases are associated, with one disease predisposing to another. These associations tend to leverage the impact of disease on the animal

Metabolic disease incidence typically increases as milk production increases and as herds become larger. The incidence of metabolic disease increases in the period commencing at calving and extending until the peak of lactation (peri-parturient period). It is characterized by dramatic changes in nutrient demand that necessitate exquisite coordination of metabolism to meet requirements for energy, glucose, minerals and amino acids by the mammary gland following calving. If the nutrient reserves are not sufficient to supply high milk production, it may further reduce them to below critical levels and clinical metabolic disease occurs. The changes may be either variation in milk secretion or sudden variation in animals feed intake because of ingestion, digestion and absorption. These variations lead to change in the internal environment of the animal.

The fact that, some dams are affected much more by these variations than others, is probably explainable on the basis of variation in internal metabolism and degree of milk production between species and individuals or even within groups of cows. This seems to invoke genetic factors, at least as predisposing cause.

Liver metabolism in late pregnancy and early lactation in dairy cows is under a great deal of stress. The metabolic demands in these periods require that the liver synthesizes more glucose from non carbohydrates precursors because the cow in these periods is often in negative energy balance, therefore, mobilization of body fat to liver during periods of negative energy balance lead to deposition of fat in the liver and fatty liver syndrome may develop. Ruminants may be prone to fatty liver because their hepatic tissue has limited capacity to export very low density lipoprotein also, a pre-partum surge of estrogen may contribute to the development of fatty liver in ruminants by increased fatty acid esterification along with limited export of triglyceride.

These factors favour the use of rigorous, quantitative monitoring of metabolic disease whenever possible. Management of the dry cow plays an important role in the control of metabolic disorders near or at calving time. Calving and the first month after freshening are critical times for the dairy cow. The major disorders affecting the fresh cow are usually the result of nutrition and feed management problems. Metabolic disorders are completely interrelated and tend to occur together

The main metabolic disorders of the fresh cow (at calving time) are:

- Milk fever
- Ketosis
- Fat cow syndrome
- Rumen acidosis
- Laminitis
- Retained placenta
- Udder edema
- Displaced abomasums.

ABBREVIATIONS

b. wt.	=	body weight
BUN	=	Blood urea nitrogen
Ca	=	Calcium
cm	=	Centimeter
Cu	=	Copper
dl	=	Deciliter
DLC	=	Differential Leukocyte Count
DM	=	Dry matter
g	=	Gram
Hb	=	Haemoglobin
I/M	=	Intramuscular
I/V	=	Intravenous
I U	=	International Unit
K	=	Potassium
Kg	=	Kilogram
l	=	Liter
mμ	=	Millimicron
MCH	=	Mean corpuscular haemoglobin
MCHC	=	Mean corpuscular haemoglobin concentration
MCV	=	Mean corpuscular volume

mEq	=	Milli equivalent
Mg	=	Magnesium
mg	=	Milligram
mm	=	Millimeter
Mn	=	Manganese
Na	=	Sodium
NaCl	=	Sodium chloride
O.D.	=	Optical density
P	=	Phosphorus
PCV	=	Packed cell volume
ppm	=	Parts per million
RBC	=	Red blood cell
Std.	=	Standard
TEC	=	Total Erythrocyte Count
TLC	=	Total Leaukocyte Count
VFAs	=	Volatile fatty acids
Zn	=	Zinc
T	=	Test
S	=	Standard
B	=	Blank

CONTENTS

Exercise 1

Clinical Examination of Sick Animals Suffering from Metabolic, Deficiency and Toxic Diseases

"Precise examination is the basis of veterinary work"

Richard Gotze

The purpose of the clinical examination is to identify the clinical abnormalities that are present and the risk factors that determine the occurrence of the disease in the individual or population. The focal point of any investigation of animal disease is the making of diagnosis and the critical part in making that decision is the clinical examination of the animal or group of animals. Without a proficient clinical examination and an accurate diagnosis it is unlikely that the treatment, control, prognosis and welfare of animals will be optimized. The level of examination set out is sufficient to enable the clinician to determine the nature of the abnormality and the system involved.

Precautions during handling of animal

The Veterinary surgeon should approach a tied-up cow from right side, assuming that this is the side from which milking is usually performed. One should not approach a cow from the left side without first patting or stroking its back. First of all veterinarian should be familiarized with the animal before going for clinical examination. It must be remembered that frightned, nervous or bad-tempered cow are liable to move suddenly side ways or kick. Cows usually kick side ways in a half circle with a slicing action.

Useful equipments for clinical examination

The veterinary surgeon should be well equipped before going for clinical examination of herd or individual animal like-

- Protective clothing's (Veterinary smock or clinical coat, apron, hand gluves etc.).
- *Instruments* : phonandoscope or stethoscope, scissors, forceps, percussion hammers, plesimeter, torch, clinical thermometer, ophthalmoscope, auriscope, urethral catheter, vaginal speculum, teat siphon, metal wedge gag, wooden mouth gag, stomach tube, nasogastric tube and probang, hoof knife, hoof tester and clipper
- *Laboratory kit* : pH paper (wide range), assorted needle and syringes, spinal needles, local anaesthetic, vessels (containers, test tubes,vials etc.) for collecting and dispatching samples.

The clinical examination of sick animals suffering from metabolic, deficiency and toxic diseases consists of recording of the history and examination of the environment and the animal.

The history should include patient data, disease history and the management history. Patient data has the accurate identification of the patient (distinguish/identification marks), species, breed, type, sex and age of the animal and owner's name and address. Disease history includes identification of present disease (the details of the clinical abnormalities observed by the owner in the sequence in which they occurred including variations in intake of food or drink, milk production, growth, respiration, defecation, urination, sweating, activity gait, posture, voice and odour), morbidity, case fatality and population mortality rates, prior treatment details, prophylactic and control measures adopted, previous exposure, transit, culling rate and previous illness. The management history includes nutrition (quantity and quality of the diet, variations in the preparation of diet), reproductive management and performance (breeding and parturition history i.e. percentage of abortion, length of breeding season, percentage of females pregnant at specified time after onset of breeding season, male/ female ratio, size and topography of breeding pastures, fertility status of females and males at breeding time, percentage of females which need assistance at parturition, percentage of newborns died at birth), Climate and general management including hygiene, adequacy of housing in terms of space, ventilation, draining, situation and suitability of troughs, opportunity for exercise and avoidance of injury to udder and other parts.

Examination of the environment is a necessary part of any clinical investigation because of the possible relationship between environmental factors and the incidence of disease. Examination of outdoor environment includes the effects of topography and soil types, population density (stocking rate), food and water supplies and waste disposal. Examination of indoor environment includes effects of housing and ventilation, level of sanitation and hygiene, measurement of population density, quality of floor, etc.

Examination of the patient animal consists of general inspection (behavior and general appearance, voice, eating, defecation, urination, posture, gait, condition and conformation), inspection of body regions (head, neck, thorax including rate, rhythm, depth and type of respiration, thorax symmetry and respiratory noises, abdomen, external genitalia, mammary gland and limbs), physical examination (palpation, percussion and auscultation) and examination of body regions (head and neck including examination of eyes, nostrils, mouth; thorax and abdomen).

Procedure: (*Source*: Text book of Veterinary Medicine by Blood *et al.*, 2000)

Record history and perform clinical examination by systematically.

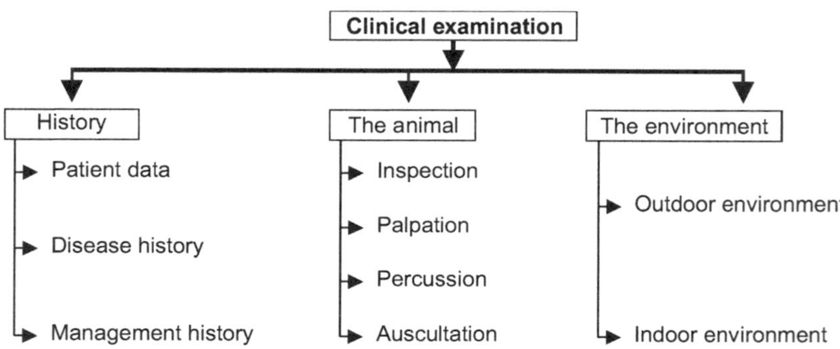

Observations

A. History

Patient data

1. Active data

Owner's name:	**Owner's address:**
Identification mark :	Age :
Species :	Sex :
Breed :	

2. Passive data- Passive data are mainly used for crompton metabolic profile test

- Passive data related to animal -
  - Date of calving :......................
  - Weight of concentrate feed/day :......................
  - Exact milk yield and mastitis status :......................
- Passive data related to herd –
  - Estimated daily forage intake :......................
  - Analysis of forage and grains :......................
  - Total herd production and number of cows in milk :......................
  - Most recent bulk milk quality data :......................

Disease history

- Present disease :......................
- Morbidity :......................
- Case fatality :......................
- Population mortality :......................
- Prior treatment :......................
- Prophylactic and control measures :......................
- Prior exposure :......................

Management history

- Nutrition history-
  - Grazing/stallfed :......................
  - Breeding history :......................

- Reproductive history
  - Percentage of abortions :.......................
  - Length of breeding season :.......................
  - % female pregnant at specified times after the onset of breeding period :.......................
  - Bull/cow ratio :.......................
  - Size and topography of breeding pasture :.......................
  - Fertility status of male and female at breeding time :.......................

B. The animal

Inspection

- General inspection
  - Behavior and general appearance : ....
  - Excitation state : ....
  - Condition and confirmation : ....
  - Posture : ....
  - Voice : ....
  - Eating : ....
  - Defecation : ....
  - Urination : ....
  - Gait : ....
- Inspection of body regions
  - Head : ....
  - Neck : ....

	Descriptor	Comments	Potential Problems
I	Intake	How much feed is being cosumed ?	Any disease : Feeding Management
N	Nose	Signs of nasal discharge, character, color, quantity	Pneumonia, Depressed attitude
S	Skin (Hair Coat)	Is the hair coat rough or smooth? Any skin lesions present?	Ketosis, LDA, RDA, Indigestion, Environment
P	Pulse	Determine heart rate and character of beat Are the jugular veins distended and pulsing	Milk fever, Toxic of septic, Heart disease, Hardware
E	Eyes	Check for discharges, lesions and ability to see.	Pneumonia, Pinkeye, Trauma
C	Condition	How does body condition compare to expected ? the herd?	High production ; Feed problems ; Disease Acidosis, Digestive diseases
T	Temperature	Determine rectal temperature	$< 100^{o}F$ = Milk fever, $> 103.5^{o}F$ = Infections, Septic or Toxic
H	Hydration	Determine fluid status - eyes, skin pinch, mouth	Septic or Toxic diseases, Digestive diseases
E	Eating Behavior	How is she eating ? Slug feeding ? Sorting the feed?	Acidosis, Digestive diseases
R	Respiration	Determine breathing rate, quality of lung sounds	Pneumonia, Bloat, Septic or Toxic diseases

R	Rumen	Assess rumen activity, gut fill	LDA, RDA, Acidosis, Indigestion, Hardware
E	Ears	Are the ears warm or cold?	Milk Fever, Septic or Toxic
F	Feces	Evaluate character, content, consistency of feces	Acidosis, Digestive diseases, Septic or Toxic diseases
U	Urine	Evaluate color, pH, ketone content of urine	Leptospirosis, Milk Fever, Ketosis
L	Legs	Presence of lessions of hoof or legs.	Footrot, Corns, Heel Wart, Laminitis
L	Lameness	How does the cow move? Obvious limps or nonuse of leg?	Laminitis, Musculoskeletal diseases
Y	Your Records	Record all cow observations and exam findings	Loss of important health information.

Source : Dairy Alliance, Pennstate University

- Thorax
  Thorax symmetry : ....
- Respiration
- Respiration rate : ....
- Respiratory rhythm : ....
- Respiratory depth : ....
- Respiratory noises : ....
- Abdomen : ....
- External genitalia : ....
- Mammary gland : ....
- Limbs : ....

Palpation

It is aimed at determining the size, consistency, temperature and sensitivity of a lesion or organ. The term used to describe palpation findings are-

- Duffy- when the structure pits on pressure as in edema.
- Firm- when structure has the consistency of normal liver
- Hard- when consistency is bone like
- Fluctuating- when the structure is soft, elastic and undulate on pressure but does not retain imprint of finger.
- Tense- when structure feels like a viscous distended with gas or fluid under some considerable pressure.
- Emphysematous- when the structure is puffy and swollen.

Percussion

In percussion the body surface is struck so as to set deep parts in the vibration and cause them to emit audible sound. The sound vary with the density of parts set in vibration and may be classified as- resonant, tympanic and dull.

C. The environment

Outdoor environment

- Effect of topography and types of soil : ....
- Stocking rate : ....
- Food supplies : ....
- Water supply and disposal : ....

Indoor environment

- Hygiene : ....
- Ventilation : ....
- Flooring : ....
- Lighting : ....

Questions

1. Examine the animals presented to you (clinically) for metabolic, deficiency and toxic diseases and interpret your results.
2. What is the posture of milk fever affected cattle?
3. What should be quality of floor for a dairy herd which helps in the prevention of downer cow syndrome?

Answer Sheet

....

....

....

....

Exercise 2

Metabolic Profile Test

Metabolic profile testing (MPT) refers to the use of a battery of tests for the diagnosis of subclinical nutritional and metabolic disease in dairy cows on a herd basis. Typically, blood samples from 5-7 animals per production group are tested for various analytes. MPT is most useful in the diagnosis and management of periparturient disease. Specific nutrient imbalances, either deficiency or excess, in the diet of late-gestation cows have been related to increased prevalence of milk fever, hypomagnesemia, retained placentas, downer cow syndrome, mastitis, udder edema, ketosis, hepatic lipidosis, and displaced abomasums.

Laboratory measurement of certain components of blood will reflect the nutritional status of the animal with or without the presence of clinical abnormalities. This gives an indication that which animals are likely to be affected with metabolic diseases.

Objectives of metabolic profile test

- This test aid in the diagnosis of nutritional imbalance and production or metabolic diseases and also as an aid in selection of superior animals.
- To explore for the methods of predicting the occurrence of the disease well in advance so that preventive measures can be considered.
- This test would theoretically be able to detect the qualitative and quantitative adequacy of the diets of cows expected to produce certain quantity of milk.
- To optimize livestock production and obtain maximum yields at minimum cost.
- In dairy animals, the major objective is to demonstrate the interrelationship between the components of blood nutrition, productivity and fertility.

Procedure

Three groups of 7 animals each are randomly selected from entire herd i.e. group I (dry cows), group II (medium yielding cows) and group III (high yielding cows). Blood should be collected three times yearly, when nutritional imbalances are most likely suspected i.e. summer, autumn and winter. Blood should preferably collect during same time for each collection with minimum excitation of cows. Five ml blood in oxalate fluoride for glucose and organic phosphorus estimation and 15 to 20 ml in heparin for estimation of rest of parameters.

Biochemical parameters-

i) Blood glucose
ii) BUN
iii) Serum inorganic phosphorus
iv) Serum Ca and Mg

v) Na and K
vi) Total protein
vii) Albumin and globulin
viii) Occasionally Cu, Fe and
ix) Plasma non-esterified fatty acids.

Haematological

i) PCV
ii) Haemoglobin (Hb)

Information to be collected during sampling

A. Related to individual animal

1. Age
2. Date of calving
3. Weight of concentrated feed per day
4. Exact milk yield and Mastitis status.

B. Related to herd

1. Estimated daily forage intake
2. Analytical data of forage and grains
3. Total herb production and number of cows in milk
4. Most recent bulk milk quality
5. Individual daily yield of six cows, particularly their peak at 3 consecutive occasions.

Merits

1. helps in determining qualitative and quantitative adequacy of diet.
2. helps in determining nutritional status of animal/herd.
3. helps in determining production/deficiency diseases in sub clinical stage.

4. helps in predicting the productivity of animal
5. helps in selecting superior quality individual.

Limitations

1. Need to be carefully planned.
2. Expensive and time consuming.
3. Sophisticated laboratory with automated analytical equipment is must.
4. Normal values are must.

Mini metabolic profile test

Blood glucose, BUN and albumin in cattle between 4-10 weeks post partum and has been recommended as a sufficient test to assess the adequacy of energy and protein intake. In this test the sampling is done at intervals of 4-6 weeks. In general the sampling should be done during early lactation and peak of lactation. It is the test used to reduce the voluminous data also to reduce the difficulty in interpretation.

Interpretation

Interpretation is difficult but the main objective should be aimed to access the inter relationship between the component of blood, nutrition, productivity and fertility.

Generally in interpretation the mean value of each parameter of each group is to be compared with mean value of the same parameter of the parent herd (which is predetermined by survey). While interpretation one should ruled out seasonal variation i.e. urea, Hb and PCV are high during summer in both lactating and non lactating cows.

Question

1. Collect and compute the data's for metabolic profile test from a herd of cows.

Answer Sheet

....

....

....

....

....

....

....

Exercise 3

Collection and Examination of Ruminal Fluid

Examination of rumen fluid was introduced for clinical diagnosis during the 1950's. The stomach of ruminant harbor beneficial microbes required for digestion of feed consumed. Stomach maintains an ideal environment (pH 6.8 to 7.2 and temperature 39-40°C) for growth and proliferation of these microfloras. In any of the ruminal disorder this homeostasis get upset resulting in shifting of microbial population (Gram negative to Gram positive) and formation and accumulation of toxic products of abnormal metabolism. This further leads to an array of pathologic process in the body. Hence physical, microbial and biochemical examination of rumen fluid can be considered as an important diagnostic tool for wide variety of disorders.

Indications

1. Diagnosis of ruminal diseases.

2. Evaluation of ruminal fluid before use in therapeutic transfusion.

Collection of rumen fluid

Rumen liquor can be collected by any of the following methods-

1. *Stomach tube* : A soft stomach tube of sufficient length depending upon the size of animal is passed to rumen very gently. It is connected to suction pump to collect the sample.

   Advantage : Non-traumatic, easy and convenient and adequate sampling.

   Disadvantage : Chances of vagal shock (rare) and restraining is required.

2. *Hypodermic needle* : sample is collected with the 6" long hypodermic needle. Needle is inserted in the lower region of triangular area on left flank particularly in young ruminants. This method is easy, safe and have the field applicability to collect the sufficient quantity of sample for clinical examination of rumen fluid

   Advantage : Less restraining is required.

   Disadvantage : Chances of peritonitis and inadequate sampling.

3. *Rumen fistula* : This method is mainly used for research purpose, there rumen fluid is collected daily at a particular interval or frequent collection. It is sort of permanent opening where rumen fistula is fixed after operating the animal on left flank and the sample is collected with the plastic tube attached with the rubber bulb.

Examination of ruminal fluid

Physical Character	Chemical Character	Microscopical examination
• Color	• pH	• Quantitative examination
• Consistency	• Methylene blue reduction test (MBRT)	• Qualitative examination
• Odor	• Cellulose digestion test	
• Sedimentation activity test	• Glucose fermentation test	
	• Nitrate reduction test	
	• Rumen fluid chloride	
	• Volatile Fatty Acids (VFA)	

Physical characters

1. Color : Depends on the diet.

   Normal :

Pure green	- In Grazing
Yellowish brown	- In straw feeding
Grey/brownish green	- Concentrate and straw feeding

   Abnormal

Dark brown/Dark green	- Simple inactivity of flora
	- Ruminal acidosis
Slightly milky	- Chronic rumen acidosis
Milky green	- Acute rumen acidosis
Greenish black	- Vagus indigestion, ruminal atony.

2. Consistency

Normal:	- Slightly viscous
Abnormal:	
Watery	- Inactive bacteria or protozoa
Excess frothy	- Frothy bloat
Semiliquid	- Vagus indigestion

3. Odor

Normal:	- Aromatic odor
Abnormal:	
Ammonia smell	- Urea poisoning
Moldy rotting	- protein putrefaction
Sour odor	- excess lactic acid/grain overfeeding
Musty/Feacal	- Vagus indigestion

4. *Sedimentation activity test* : The principal of this test is that in fresh and healthy rumen fluid gas is produced due to microbial fermentation which causes fibrous material to float. Normally most of the fine food particles (and infusoria) begin to settle at once, while the larger and more fibrous constituents are carried upwards by gas bubbles resulting from fermentation, forming a broad, foamy upper layer. The time required for the completion of sedimentation and flotation is measured, and is referred to as the sediment activity time (SAT).

Procedure

1. Take 20 ml freshly collected and sieved rumen liquor in a test tube.
2. Record the time taken for sedimentation/floatation.

Interpretation

1. Normal SAT in cattle - 4-8 minutes.
2. No appreciable sedimentation/floatation - Vagal indigestion/frothy bloat
3. Rapid sedimentation and no floatation (SAT <3 min) - Severe lactacidosis/inactive microflora
4. Acid and alkaline indigestion and non-specific anorexia- 9 to 15 min.

Sedimentation Activity Test
(Evaluation of microfloral activity)

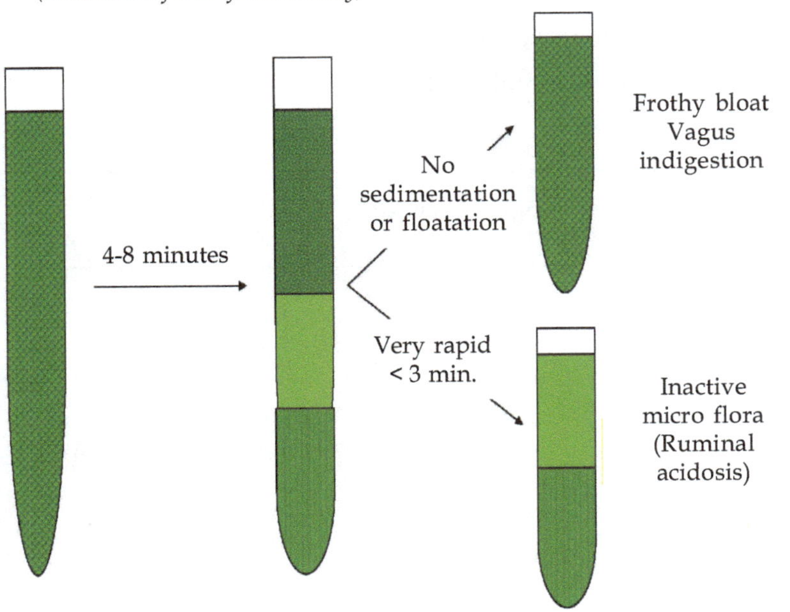

In Normal

Fine food particles - begin to settle at once

Larger & more fibrous *Particles* - carried upward forming broad upper layer

Chemical characters

1. Hydrogen ion concentration (pH)

Normal :- Ranged between 6.8 to 7.2

Abnormal

Elevated pH (Rumen alkalosis)-upto 8.5

- Simple indigestion
- Urea poisoning
- Putrefaction of ruminal content
- Protein intake

Lowered pH (Rumen acidosis) - 4.0-5.5

- Grain overfeeding
- Chronic ruminal acidosis

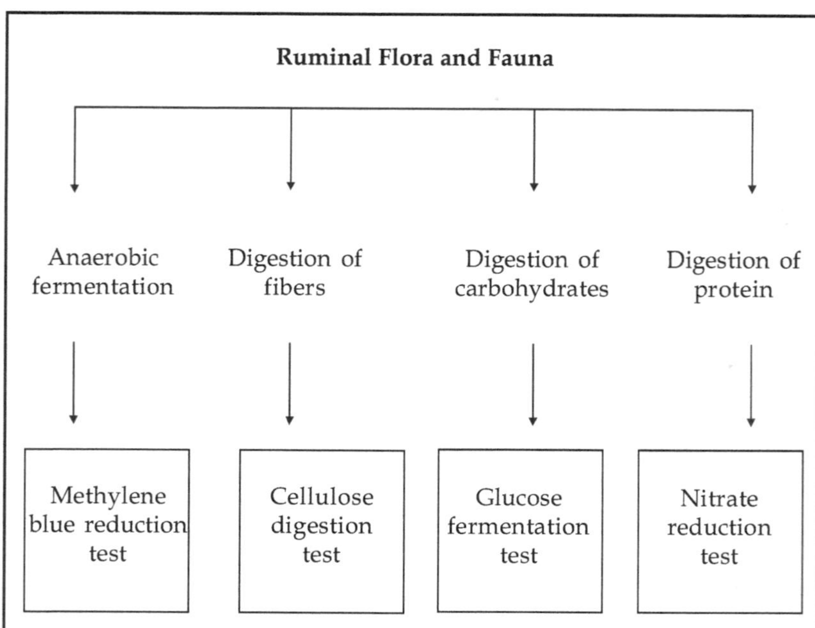

2. Methylene blue reduction test (MBRT)

This test measure redox potential of rumen liquor to asses the microbial status of rumen fluid.

Procedure

1. Take 20 ml of sieved rumen liquor in two test tube.
2. Add 1 ml of 0.03% methylene blue solution in a test tube and another test tube use as control and mix properly.
3. Incubate the tube at 37°C and record the time required to decolorize.

Interpretation

Normal active microflora	- Colour disappear within 3-4 minutes.
Inappetance and Inactive flora	- >15 mins
Rumen acidosis	- <5 mins. Above pH 5.2
	- >5 mins. Below pH 5.2
Hydrochloric acidosis	- >5 mins.

3. Cellulose digestion test

To asses the ability of cellulolytic microflora to produce the enzymes responsible for the digestion of feed/fodder (cellulose) material.

Procedure

1. Take 10 ml of sieved rumen fluid in a test tube.
2. Add 0.3 ml of 16% glucose solution.
3. Put a thread of pure cellulose (free from synthetic fibers, e.g. cotton wool) in the test tube in the lower end the thread needs to be weighted with a glass bead or other weight.
4. Incubate the test tube at 37°C.
5. Record the time required to digest the cellulose thread.

Interpretation

Fully active rumen fluid will digest the cellulose within 30 to 48 hours to such an extent that the weight will fall to the bottom of the tube. In case of any ruminal disorder this time of digestion will increase.

4. Glucose fermentation test

The ability of the microflora to break down (ferment) glucose is measured indirectly from the volume of gas formed.

Procedure

1. Take 10 ml of sieved rumen fluid in a beaker.
2. Add 0.5 ml of 16% glucose solution.
3. Mix both and place the mixture in a fermentation saccharometer.
4. Incubate at 37°C.
5. Result is read after 30 and 60 minutes.

Interpretation

1-2 ml gas/hour	- Active microflora
No gas	- Inactive microflora, acute rumen acidosis
Decreased gas	- Rumen decomposition, Rumenal alkalosis
Normal/increased gas	- Latent rumen acidosis
Increased gas	- Frothy bloat

5. Nitrite reduction test

This test provides information on the activity of microbes that degradate and synthesize nitrogenous compounds.

Procedure

1. Take 10 ml of sieved rumen fluid in three test tubes.
2. Add 0.2, 0.5 or 0.7 ml of 0.025% potassium nitrite solution in three test tubes.
3. All test tubes transferred to a water bath at 39°C.
4. At every five minutes one drop from each tube is placed in the small wells of a ceramic plate.
5. Add 2 drops of reagent I (2 ml of sulfanilic acid in 30% acetic acid to make 200 ml) and 2 drops of reagent II (0.6 ml alpha-naphthylamine, 16 ml concentrated acetic acid, 140 ml distilled water) in the wells of ceramic plate.
6. Record the disappearance of red color at different time intervals. Samples that still contain nitrite are colored red.

Interpretation

With fluid from cattle fed a mixed ration, nitrite should disappear after 5-10 minutes in tube 1, 20 minutes in tube 2 and 30 minutes in tube 3. Reduction is more rapid when the cattle are fed green fodder or have ruminal decomposition or bloat, and slower when a deficient ration is fed, or when the animal lacks appetite. In case of lactacidosis no reduction even after 45 mins.

Microscopic examination

Microbial examination

The rumen microorganisms can be divided into three main groups: the bacteria, the protozoa and the fungi. Smear made of ruminal fluid is dried, fixed as stained by Gram's stain. Gram positive organism will show violet colour while Gram negative organisms will show red or pink colour. In case of ruminal lactoacidosis there is predominance of Gram positive bacteria e.g. *Streptococcus bovis, Lactobacilli.*

Bacterial count

- Sieved rumen fluid is centrifuged at 3000 rpm for 5 min.
- Mix 10% formalin in the ratio of 1:1 to kill bacteria and strain rumen fluid.
- Dilution of formalized ruminal fluid is made at the level of 1:10, 1:100, 1:1000 with distilled water.
- Take 0.01 ml of diluted sample on 2 x 2 cm area of a clean glass slide and spread evenly and allowed to dry on hot plate.
- After drying stain it with Gram's stain.
- Examin under the oil immersion lens of microscope by using 10x eye piece. A total of 30 to 50 fields are counted. The count per g or ml of ruminal fluid is to be calculated by multiplying the average of fields with the factor (microscopic factor) obtained by calibrating the microscope with certain set of ocular (X 10) using oil immersion.

Protozoal motility

A drop of fresh ruminal fluid is taken on a clear glass slide and cover slip is placed over it and examined under low power microscope and graded as follows:

Motility	Activity
• Highly motile and very crowded	+++
• Motile and crowded	++
• Sluggish motility and low numbers	+
• No or sporadic alive fauna	0

Moderate (+ +) to vigorous (+++) indicate normal protozoal activity. Ratio of live : dead protozoa should be noted for clinical purpose. Presence of large and medium ciliates in large number indicate active rumen fluid, while only small ciliates are present indicate the forestomach indigestion. In acute ruminal acidosis all protozoa are dead.

Protozoal count

Reagents

- Formal saline (0.85% normal saline and formalin in equal volume)
- 5% Lugol's iodine.
- 30% Glycerine.

Working solution

Formal saline	-	1.0 ml
Lugol's iodine (5%)	-	2.5 ml
Glycerine (30%)	-	1.5 ml

At first 1:10 dilution of freshly collected rumial fluid is done with working solution. Then following a gentle shaking 0.1 ml is placed in a counting slide with a pipette and covered with cover glass 1000 mm^2 (5 x 2 cm). Differential total counts are carried out by very low power objectives. A total of 30-50 fields are to be counted. Average count is taken as number of protozoa/mm^2. Multiplying the average count by the number of fields on counting slide will give protozoal count in 0.1 ml of diluted sample.

Total protozoa/ml of rumen liquor =
Avg. protozoa counted X Vol. of sample X dilution

Protozoal count may be graded as plenty (+ + +), moderate (+ +), few (+) and none (-). Number of protozoa may decrease due to poor quality ration and starvation. It is increased when the cattle is properly fed with adequate ration.

Observations and Interpretation

Questions

1. Collect and evaluate the rumen fluid from the given animal.
2. Write the pH of normal ruminal fluid and in different digestive dysfunction.
3. Write the predominant ruminal microorganisms in alkaline and chronic indigestion respectively.
4. Write the name and importance of VFAs.

Answer Sheet

....

....

....

....

....

....

Exercise 4

Collection of Blood and Blood Serum and Evaluation of Haemogram for Metabolic Profile Test

The main aim of blood testing is to ascertain the adequacy of each new diet in relation to the herd's requirements, *i.e. what the cows think of their rations*. So blood sampling should be carried out as soon as possible after major changes in dietary constituents. But two weeks must elapse after the changes to allow the rumen to become fully adapted. The metabolic profile is based on the concept that the laboratory measurement of certain components of the blood will reflect the nutritional status of the animal with or without the manifestation of clinical abnormalities. The values of Hb, PCV, TEC, TLC, DLC and erythrocytic indices are useful indicator of health status of the animal.

Timing of blood collection

1. Blood sampling should be carried out as soon as possible after major changes in dietary constituents.

2. Typical blood sampling times are two to three weeks after: Winter housing, change of silage, start of maize silage, change of cake, turn out, blood test prompted by dietary changes, start of block calving. Other useful times are: At autumn grass, dry cows at grass, during summer grazing, when there are specific problems - in which case act quickly.

The Sites of Collection

Venous blood collected from the following site with the help of hypodermic needle and is used for analysis.

Site of collection	Advantages/Comments	Disadvantages
Cattle		
+++ Jugular vein	Large volume collected	Risk to collector
++ Coccygeal vein	Handling ease	Small volumes
+ Cephalic vein	Possibly easier in a calf	-
Sheep		
+++ Jugular Vein	Moderate to large volume collected	- Animal needs to be well resieved.
+++ Cephalic Vein	Small volume collected	-
++ Lateral Saphenous vein	Small volume collected	-
Goat		
+++ Jugular vein	Convenient	
+ Cephalic vein		
Horse		
+++ Jugular vein	Convenient Large volume collected	
Pig		
+++ Cranial Vena Cava	Large volume requires.	Specialised restraining techniques requires
++ Marginal Ear Vein	Small volume collected	Requires sedation
++ Jugular Vein	Moderate volume (10ml)	
Dog		
+++ Cephalic Vein	Small to moderate amounts of blood collected.	
+++ Jugular	Large volume of collected	
++ Medial Saphenous Vein	Small to moderate amounts of blood collected.	
+ Femoral Vein	Small to moderate amounts of blood collected.	

+++ Preferred Method
++ Acceptable Method
+ Possible Method

All equipments employed for collecting blood sample must be clean, dry and sterile. In general, plasma or serum should be harvested as soon as possible after blood collection.

Anticoagulants

Choice of anticoagulants depends upon the type of examination to be carried out.

Anticoagulant	Concentration	Use
EDTA	1-2 mg/ ml of blood	Haematology, thrombocyte count, total protein, BUN, plasma fibrinogen, enzymology etc.
Heparin	0.2 mg/ ml of blood	Haematocrit study, blood gas analysis, biochemical and mineral analysis etc.
Sodium fluoride	2.5 mg/ ml of blood	Excellent for blood glucose study

Collection of blood sample

1. Remove the hairs at the site of blood collection by shaving for proper visualization of concerned vein.
2. Clean the skin with 70% alcohol or other antiseptics.
3. Raise the vein by pressure of thumb or finger. Rubbing the site with alcohol which helps in outlining the veins more clearly.
4. Insert the sterilized needle into vein.
5. Gently aspirate the blood with syringe to avoid collapse of the vein.
6. Withdraw the needle from vein. Before withdrawing the needle, release your hold on the vein.
7. Mix the blood gently but do not shake vigorously to avoid rupturing of RBCs.

Collection of Plasma

Take the blood sample in a small test tube, centrifuge it at 3000 rpm for 10 minutes. Remove the tube & observe the contents.

The blood cells can be seen packed at the bottom of the tube below a clear plasma fluid. Siphon off the plasma carefully and preserve the same in storage vial. In case of the haemolysis repeat the process right from blood collection.

Collection of Serum

Take 5 ml of freshly drawn blood in a test tube without adding anticoagulants. Place the test tube in slanting position and allow it to clot at room temperature. Let the clotted blood to stand for 15 minutes preferably in a refrigerator. The blood clot will retract and clear fluid will ooze out. Remove the supernatant serum carefully. For quicker results, the clotted blood may be centrifuged for 15 minutes for 2500 rpm.

Observations

Erythrocyte sedimentation rate ....mm/hour

Packed cell volume .... %

Haemoglobin .... g%

Total erythrocyte count .... $\times 10^{12}$ /l

Total leukocyte count .... $\times 10^{9}$ /l

Differential leukocyte count

Relative count (%)

Absolute count ($\times 10^{9}$ /l)

MCV ....

MCH ....

MCHCK ....

Interpretation

Questions

1. Collect the blood and perform haemogram from the given animal.
2. Write the normal haematological values of dairy cattle, goat, sheep, horse and pig.
3. What is absolute count? How will you calculate absolute neutrophils count from relative count?
4. Which is the best for biochemical analysis weather plasma or serum?

Answer Sheet

....

....

....

....

....

....

....

....

Exercise 5

Estimation of Blood Glucose for Computing Metabolic Profile Test

Carbohydrates are constituents of all living cells. Animal as well as plant cells use carbohydrates as source of energy. Blood glucose is a useful indicator of energy metabolism and fertility status. Under certain clinical circumstances, estimation of carbohydrates becomes essential. Sugar levels (particularly glucose) in blood or urine are used as an important parameter for diagnosis of ketosis and diabetes mellitus.

Principle

At 100°C in the presence of glacial acetic acid glucose reacts with O-toluidine to form N-glucosylamine giving blue-green colour. The color intensity is measured at 630 nm spectrophotometrically.

Reagent

1. *O-tuluidine reagent* : Dissolve 1.5 g of thiourea in about 300 ml of glacial acetic acid. Add 9.5 g sodium borate

and dissolve. Add 80 ml of O-toluidine and make the volume to 1 litre with acetic acid.

2. *Trichloroacetic acid 3%.* : 3 gm trichloroacetic acid is dissolved in distilled water to make the final volume 100 ml.

3. Standard glucose solution (0.1mg / ml) in 0.1% benzoic acid which acts as a preservative).

Method (O-Toluidine method)

There are two procedures

A. Direct method

This method is applied for clear unhaemolysed plasma or serum.

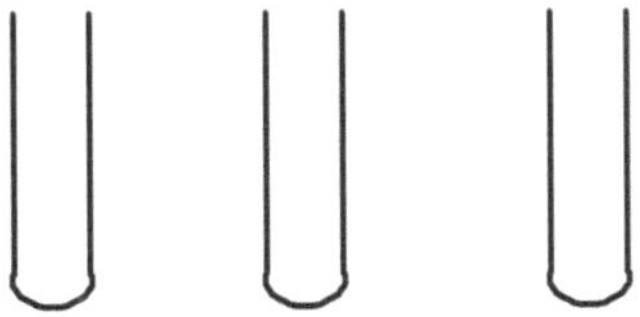

	T	S	B
1. Serum sample	0.1 ml	-	-
2. Sugar standard	-	0.1 ml	-
3. Distilled water	-	-	0.1 ml
4. O-toluidine reagent	4.0 ml	4.0 ml	4.0 ml

5. Mix and place the tubes in boiling water bath for 15 min.
6. Cool in tap water and read OD of test and standard at 630 nm against blank using spectrophotometer.

B. Indirect method

This method is used for haemolysed plasma, or serum or whole blood.

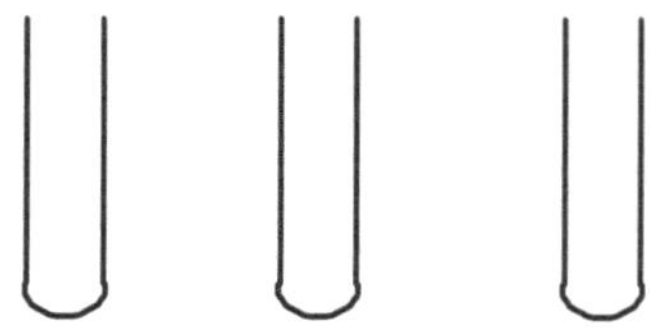

		T	S	B
1.	Trichloroacetic acid (3%)	0.9 ml	0.9 ml	0.9 ml
2.	Serum sample	0.1 ml	-	-
3.	Sugar standard	-	0.1 ml	-
4.	Distilled water	-	-	0.1 ml
	Centrifuge all tubes at 1500 rpm for 15 min and remove supernatant			
5.	O-toluidine reagent	4.0 ml	4.0 ml	4.0 ml
6.	Supernatant of corresponding tube	0.2 ml	0.2 ml	0.2 ml

7. Mix and place the tubes in boiling water bath for 15 min.
8. Cool in tap water and read OD of test and standard at 630 nm against blank using spectrophotometer.

Calculation

$$\text{Plasma/ Serum / Blood glucose (mg/dl)} = \frac{\text{O.D. of Test}}{\text{O.D. of Standard}} \text{ X conc. of Std.}$$

Result : Concentration of sugar in plasma/ serum/ blood is _______ mg/dl.

Interpretation

Questions

1. Estimate the glucose level in given sample.
2. Write the normal values of blood glucose in different species of animals.
3. Enlist the important livestock diseases in which hyper and hypoglycemia develops.
4. Discuss relationship of blood glucose with prevention of metabolic disorders.
5. Which type of fluid therapy should be preferred in the case of ketosis in dairy cattle?

Answer Sheet

....

....

....

....

....

....

....

....

....

....

....

....

....

Exercise 6

Blood Glucose Tolerance Test (GTT) for Computing Metabolic Profile Test

The glucose is utilized in the body for immediate energy requirements. The utilization of glucose depends on the integrated activity of digestive system metabolism and endocrine system of the body. Glucose tolerance is referred as the capacity of animal to regulate elevated blood glucose on ingestion or infusion, gradually. The level of glucose that can be tolerated by an animal without producing glucosurea is indicative of tolerance. Glucose load challenges the pancreas to release insulin which in turn regulates blood glucose level. If the insulin release is adequate and target cells have healthy receptors, elevated blood glucose level return to base value within 2 hours and glucose does not appear in urine. An increased glucose tolerance means limited rise and rapid fall in blood glucose in short span than the normal rate of utilization.

Procedure

The glucose tolerance test is of 2 types: Oral glucose tolerance test (OGTT) and Intravenous glucose tolerance test (IGTT). The oral route is chosen for non ruminants and intravenous route for ruminants and animals having alimentary dysfunction.

1. Oral Glucose Tolerance Test

The test in animals can be performed as described below -

1. The animal is fasted for at least 24 hours prior to the test.
2. Collect blood sample for fasting blood sugar level.
3. Give glucose 1g/Kg body weight in little water, orally.
4. Collect blood sample at 30, 60, 120, 180 and 240 minutes after glucose administration.
5. Collect the plasma by centrifuging the tube at 2000 rpm for 10 minutes and estimate glucose.
6. Plot the graph between blood glucose level (mg %) and time (hours).
7. If the animal is non diabetic, the level of glucose will not rise above 160 mg/dl at the end of first hour and will return to normal by the end of second hour. In non diabetic animals fasting blood sugar level is less than 110 mg/dl. If animal is diabetic, the glucose level will be higher than 150 mg/dl at the end of first hour and it will not return to normal within 2 hours.

2. Intravenous Glucose Tolerance Test

1. The animal is fed carbohydrate rich diet for 3 days and then it is kept on fast for at least 16 hours prior to the test.
2. The blood sample is collected for fasting blood sugar level.

3. At the rate of 0.5 g/Kg body weight glucose is administered intravenously as 50% sterile glucose within 30 seconds in large animal it can be completed within 2-3 minutes.
4. The blood sample is collected at 5, 15, 30, 45, 60 and 120 minutes after the infusion.
5. Collect the plasma by centrifuging the tube at 2000 rpm for 10 minutes and estimate glucose.
6. Plot the graph on semi log between blood glucose levels (mg/dl) and time (hours) and calculate glucose half life or turn over rate.

In non diabetic animal the blood glucose level returns to normal level within 90 minutes.

Observation

Blood glucose at different time intervals-

Interpretation

Questions

1. Perform a blood glucose tolerance test in given animal
2. Which blood anticoagulant should be used in glucose tolerance test?
3. Write the name of diseases of animals in which glucose tolerance test should be performed.

Answer Sheet

Exercise 7

Estimation of Blood Urea Nitrogen for Computing Metabolic Profile Test

Urea is the detoxification product of the ammonia derived from the deamination of amino acids. Urea is therefore the most common nitrogen-containing end product of protein catabolism. Its synthesis from ammonia occurs in the liver (via the urea cycle), and it is then excreted by the kidneys. The concentration of urea inside red cells is slightly less than in plasma due to the presence of large amounts of hemoglobin inside the cells. Whole blood urea concentration is therefore slightly less than plasma (or serum) urea. Therefore, usually serum is used instead of whole blood for the determination of urea. The familiar term BUN (blood urea nitrogen) persists in spite of the fact that it is serum urea nitrogen which is usually measured.

Blood urea nitrogen is an important component of metabolic profile test, can be applied as an adjunct in diagnosis. It was found to show the wide variation among the animal's population. Its levels have been found to be influenced by physiological states of animals and season. In most clinical situations, changes in urea levels are more dependent upon kidney function than upon liver function. Increased urea levels are associated with renal diseases as well as dehydration, diabetic coma, hypoadrenal crisis, gastrointestinal haemorrhage and circulatory collapse. Decreased values are observed in some cases of severe liver diseases.

Principle

Urea reacts with diacetyl monoxime in acidic medium at 95°C - 100°C to give pink colored complex. Ferric ions are used to oxidize hydroxylamine formed in the reaction. Absorbance of pink end product is measured at 520+ 15 nm. The intensity of color developed is proportional to the conc. of urea present in the specimen.

Reagents

1. *Diacetyl monoxime* : 1.56 g diacetyl monoxime in 250 ml distilled water.
2. *Thiosemicarbazide* : 41 mg thiosemicarbazide in 250 ml distilled water. Keep in brown bottle.
3. *Ferric chloride reagent* : 324 mg ferric chloride in 10 ml of 56% orthophosphoric acid. Keep in brown bottle.
4. *20% Sulphuric acid(V/V)* : Take 20 ml concentrated sulphuric acid in distilled water and make final volume to 100 ml.
5. *Acid reagent* : To 1000 ml of 20% sulphuric acid, add 1 ml of ferric chloride reagent.
6. *10% Trichloroacetic acid* : Dissolve 10 mg trichloroacetic acid in distilled make the volume to 100 ml.

7. *Preservative diluent for standard* : Dissolve 40 mg phenyl mercuric acetate in about 250 ml distilled water with heating. Transfer the solution into a measuring cylinder. Add 0.3 ml of concentarted sulphuric acid and make the volume to 1litre with water.

8. *Standard urea*- 10 mg urea in one liter of preservative diluents (1 ml = 0.01 mg).

Method

(Diacetyl Monoxime Method: Richter, H.J. & Lapointe, Y.S. 1962. *Clin. Chem.* 8:335)

Preparation of supernatant- Take 3.4 ml of dist. water in a centrifuge tube, add 0.1 ml blood. Mix. add 1.5 ml of 10% trichloroacetic acid and mix. Left for 5 minutes. Centrifuge it, collect the supernatant.

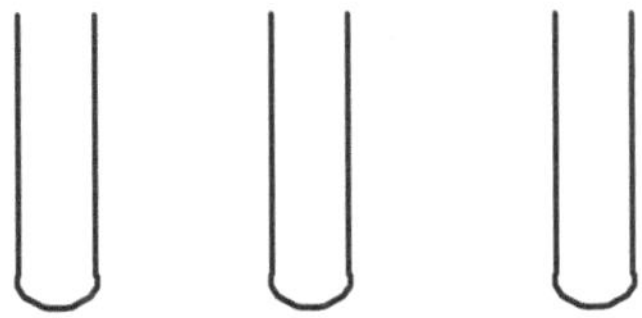

	T	S	B
1. Blood supernatant	1.0 ml	-	-
2. Urea standard	-	1.0 ml	-
3. Distilled water	-	-	1.0 ml
4. Diacetyl monoxime reagent	1.0 ml	1.0 ml	1.0 ml
5. Thiosemicarbazide	1.0 ml	1.0 ml	1.0 ml
6. Acid reagent	3.0 ml	3.0 ml	3.0 ml

7. Mix and place the tubes in boiling water bath for 15 min.

8. Cool in tap water and read OD of test and standard at 540 nm against blank using spectrophotometer.

Calculation

$$\text{Urea (mg / 100 ml of blood)} = \frac{\text{O.D of Unknown}}{\text{O. D. of standard}} \times 0.01 \times \frac{100}{0.02}$$

Result : The blood contains urea .... mg / dl.

Interpretation

Questions

1. Estimate the BUN in given sample.
2. Write normal values of BUN in different species of animals.
3. Write relationship between BUN and serum creatinin.
4. Write the diseases of dairy animals in which BUN level increased.

Answer Sheet

....

....

....

....

....

....

Exercise 8

Estimation of Serum Calcium, Magnesium and Inorganic Phosphorus for Computing Metabolic Profile Test

The levels of calcium (Ca), inorganic phosphorus (P) and magnesium (Mg) may help in early diagnosis of metabolic and deficiency disorders and for monitoring the herd health status of dairy cattle to maintain production and reproduction.

Estimation of Serum calcium

Calcium is present in 2 forms - inorganic and organic forms. Most of the functions of the calcium depend upon the ionized form. For estimation of serum calcium the most commonly used method is Clark and Collip method.

Principle

Calcium is precipitated by reacting serum with ammonium oxalate. The excess of oxalate is removed by washing with ammonia and then treated with sulphuric acid to convert calcium oxalate into oxalic acid. Then, it is titrated with standard potassium permanganate.

Reagents

1. *Ammonium oxalate, 4%:* Dissolve 4 g ammonium oxalate in distilled water to make the final volume 100 ml.
2. *Ammonia, 2%:* Take 2 ml ammonia in distilled water to make the final volume 100 ml.
3. *Sulphuric acid, 1N*: Take 28 ml concentrated sulphuric acid and make the final volume 1000 ml with distilled water.
4. *Stock potassium permanganate, 0.1N*: Dissolve 3.16 g potassium permanganate in distilled water to make the final volume 1000 ml.
5. *Potassium permanganate, 0.01N*: Add 10 ml potassium permanganate stock solution in 90 ml distilled water.
6. *Sodium oxalate, 0.01N*: Dissolve 0.67 g ammonium oxalate in distilled water to make the final volume 1000 ml.

Procedure: (Clark and Collip method)

1. Take 2 ml of serum and add 2ml water and 1ml of 4% ammonium oxalate in a centrifuge tube. Mix thoroughly and centrifuge at 1,500 rpm for 15 minutes.
2. Pour off supernatant fluid and filter by inverting on filter paper for few minutes.
3. Dissolve the filtrate by mixing 2ml of 1N sulphuric acid and shake vigorously. Keep the tube in water bath until precipitate completely dissolves.
4. Titrate the solution while it is hot with 0.01N potassium permanganate until a pink color develop and persist for at least for 1 minute.

5. Note the volume of 0.01N potassium permanganate used.
6. For preparation of blank take 2ml of 1N sulphuric acid and titrate it with 0.01N potassium permanganate.

Calculation

Suppose the volume of 0.01N potassium permanganate is *x* ml. and, the volume of 1N potassium permanganate is *y* ml.

$$\text{Serum calcium (mg/100ml)} = \frac{(x-y) \times 0.2 \times 100}{2}$$

$$= (x-y) \times 10$$

Result : The concentration of serum calcium in given sample is _______mg/100ml.

Estimation of serum magnesium : (Titan yellow method)

Principle

Proteins of the serum are precipitated by sodium tungustate and H_2SO_4 combination. The magnesium in a protein free filtrate is complexed with titan yellow (a dye) in an alkaline medium resulting red colouration which is measured by colorimeter.

Reagents

1. *Sodium tungstate solution, 10% (w/v)* : 10 gm sodium tungstate in 100 ml distilled water.
2. *H_2SO_4, 2/3 N* : 18.8 ml concentrated H_2SO_4 and make final volume upto 1 liter with distilled water.
3. *Polyvinyl alcohol, 0.05% (w/v)* : With the aid of gentle heat dissolve 0.125 gm of polyvinyl alcohol in distilled water, cool and dilute to 250 ml.
4. *Titan yellow, 0.05% (w/v)* : Dissolve 0.05 gm of titan yellow in distill water and dilute to exactly 100 ml. The stock solution is stable in a dark bottle for weeks. A working standard solution containing 0.015% of titan yellow is made fresh every few days by diluting 3 ml of stock solution with 7 ml of distilled water.
5. *Calcium chloride solution* : 16.13 mg of Calcium chloride in 100 ml of distilled water.
6. *Sodium hydroxide, 4N* : Dissolve 160 gm of sodium hydroxide in water, cool and dilute to 1 liter.
7. *Stock standard of Magnesium* : 8.458 gm Magnesium chloride dissolve in distilled water and make final volume upto 1 liter with distilled water.
8. *Working standard of Magnesium* : Dilute 1 ml of stock standard to 200 ml with distilled water.

Procedure

Preparation of protein free filtrate (PFF) : Take 1 ml serum, 5 ml distilled water, 2 ml sodium tungstate and 2 ml 2/3 N H_2SO_4, into a test tube. Mix the contents and filter it, filtrate is called protein free filtrate.

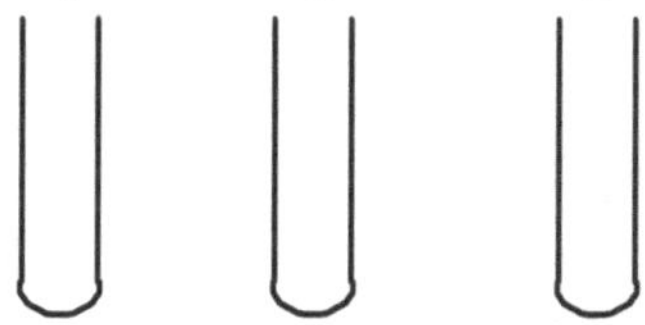

		T	S	B
1.	PFF	5.0 ml	-	-
2.	Working standard	-	1.0 ml	-
3.	Calcium chloride	-	-	1.0 ml
4.	Distilled water	1.0 ml	5.0 ml	5.0 ml
5.	Polyvinyl alcohol	1.0 ml	1.0 ml	1.0 ml
6.	Titan yellow	1.0 ml	1.0 ml	1.0 ml
7.	NaOH	2.0 ml	2.0 ml	2.0 ml

8. Wait for 1 minute and read the optical density of sample and standard at 540 mm wave length using green filter.

Calculation

$$\text{mg of Mg/100 ml of serum} = \frac{\text{O. D. of sample}}{\text{O. D. of Standard}} \times 0.02 \times 100$$

Here

0.02 - working standard solution contains 0.02 mg of Mg/ml of sample.

100 - Dilution factor.

Result : The concentration of serum calcium in given sample is _______mg/100ml.

Estimation of serum inorganic phosphorus : (Taussky and Shorr method)

Principle

A trichloroacetic acid filtrate is treated with ammonium molybdate solution, which combines with phosphate to form phosphomolybdate. The molybdate thus formed is reduced with ferrous sulfate and the blue color produced is measured photometrically and is proportional to the amount of phosphorus originally present.

Reagents

1. *Trichloroacetic acid, 12% (w/v)* : Dissolve 120 gm of trichloroacetic acid in water and dilute to exactly 1 liter.
2. *Trichloroacetic acid, 34% (w/v) :* Dissolve 340 gm of trichloroacetic acid in water and dilute to exactly 1 liter.
3. *Sulfuric acid, 10N* : Add slowly to about 700 ml of distilled water 278 ml of concentrated sulphuric acid. Cool and dilute to 1 liter with distilled water.
4. *Ammonium molybdate, stock solution, 10%* : Add 50 gm of $(NH_4)_6 Mo_7 O_{24.} 4H_2$ liter beaker and add 400 ml of 10N sulphuric acid with constant stirring to prevent caking. When completely dissolved, transfer the solution to a 500 ml volumetric flask and wash in quantitatively with 10N sulphuric acid to the mark.
5. *Ferrous sulfate ammonium (molybdate reagent stock)* : Prepare just prior to using. Transfer 10 ml of ammonium molybdate solution to a 100 ml volumetric flask and dilute to about 70 ml. Add 5 gm of $FeSO_4$ $7H_2O$ make upto volume with water and shake until the crystal are dissolved. Transfer to a brown glass bottle.

Method

1. To a test tube containing 3.5 ml of 12% trichloroacetic acid and 0.20 ml of serum, mix and allow to stand for 10 min. and then centrifuge rapidly for 10 min. Include a blank containing 0.20 ml distill water and 3 ml of 12% trichloroacetic acid.
2. Transfer 3 ml of the clear supernatant filtrate to a cuvette and add 2 ml of ferrous sulfate molybdate reagent.
3. After 1 min (or within 2 hours) read the unknown against the blank at a wave length of 660 mm using the red filter.
4. Prepare calibration curve of different concentration of standard and determine the concentration of phosphorus as mg/dl of serum.

Standardization

Prepare a stock standard solution by dissolving 0.1196 gm of anhydrous potassium dihydrogen phosphate in water and diluting to exactly 100 ml. this solution is stored in refrigerator. Two working standard solutions containing respectively, the equivalent of 5 and 10 mg phosphorous per 100 ml of serum are prepared by appropriate dilution and acidification of the aqueous stock standard solution in the following way: Dilute 1 to 2 ml of the stock standard solution to exactly 100 ml with 11.5% (w/v) trichloroacetic acid. These solutions are stable for about 3 weeks when kept in a refrigerator. Exactly 3 ml aliquots of these working standard solutions are analyzed by the same procedure that is used for serum filtrates (step 2 & 3). Record the A or % T and prepare a calibration table or curve as desired.

Observations

Ca ....

Mg ....

P ....

Interpretation

Questions

1. Write normal values of serum Ca, Mg and inorganic P in domestic animals.
2. What is the role of Ca supplementation during last trimester of pregnancy in occurrence of milk fever in dairy cattle?
3. What is the importance of Ca, Mg and P in relation with metabolic diseases?
4. Write the normal ratio of Ca:P in blood. How this ratio is maintained in blood?

Answer Sheet

....

....

....

....

....

....

Exercise 9

Estimation of Serum Sodium, Potassium for Computing Metabolic Profile Test

Sodium and potassium are the most important electrolytes of the body fluid. The sodium as sodium chloride is contained in body fluids. The potassium is also essential in body fluids and its concentration is controlled by the kidneys. The estimation of sodium-potassium balance makes an important contribution as component of metabolic profile test. Low level of Na occurs in early lactation of low grazing on summer pasture and also increasing age, depraved appetite, polydipsia and polyurea.

Reagents

1. *Sodium standards* : Dissolved 5.85 gm of dried sodium chloride in 1 liter with triple glass distilled water. This serves as stock solution and contains 100 mEq of sodium/ liter.

Working standard are prepared from the above stock solution by measuring 10, 11, 12, 13, 14, 15, 16, 17, 18, 19 and 20 ml aliquots into 1 liter volumetric flasks and is diluted to the mark with triple glass distilled water. These standards represent 100, 110, 120, 130, 140, 150, 160, 170, 180, 190 and 200 mEq of sodium/liter at 1:100 dilutions.

2. *Potassium standards* : Dissolved 0.746 gm of potassium chloride in distilled water in 1 liter volumetric flask. The volume is made upto mark with triple glass distilled water. This solution serves as stock solution and contains 10 mEq of potassium/liter.

   Working standard solution equivalent to 30, 31, 32, 33, 34, 35, and upto 50 mEq of potassium/liter at a dilution rate of 1:100 are prepared by diluting respectively 30, 31, 32, 33, 34, 35 and 50 ml of stock solution to 1 liter mark in a volumetric flasks with triple distilled water.

Method (Burriel Marti and Ramirez Munoz, 1957)

1. The serum/plasma diluted in ratio of 1:100 with triple glass distilled water.
2. A calibration/standard curve is prepared by reading each of the standards in the flame photometer.
3. The unknowns are read in flame photometer, using sodium/potassium filter.
4. The value of serum sodium and potassium are expressed in mEq/liter.

Observations

Na (mEq/liter)

K (mEq/liter)

Interpretation

Questions

1. Estimate the Na and K in given samples.
2. Write normal serum concentrations of Na and K in different domestic animals.
3. Write management practices for correction of acute and chronic deficiency of these elements in ruminants.
4. What is the importance of Na and K in metabolic profile test in high yielder dairy cows?

Answer Sheet

....

....

....

....

....

....

....

....

....

Exercise 10

Estimation of Serum Total Proteins, Albumin and Globulin for Computing Metabolic Profile Test

Total protein: (Biuret method)

There are several methods of estimating protein, in food, agricultural and clinical samples, each of them varying in sensitivity and applicability.

Principle

Biuret method is highly specific for protein and is based on the formation of the blue peptide-copper complex in alkaline solution. It is a method of choice in the clinical laboratory because of the simplicity accuracy and precision. The major limitation of the method is its poor sensitivity for many dilute solutions. The principle of this method is that the peptide bonds in protein react with biuret reagent to give a violet colored complex known as cupric potassium biuret. The colour intensity of which is proportional to protein concentration.

Reagents

1. *Protein standard (5 mg/ml BSA, Bovine serum albumin)* : It should be prepared fresh or just before of use.
2. *Biuret reagent :* The reagent is prepared by dissolving 3 g of copper sulphate and 9 g of Rochelle's salt (sodium potassium tartarate) in 500 ml of 0.2 N sodium hydroxide solutions. To this solution is added 5 g of potassium iodide and volume made up to 1000 ml with 0.2N sodium hydroxide.

Procedure

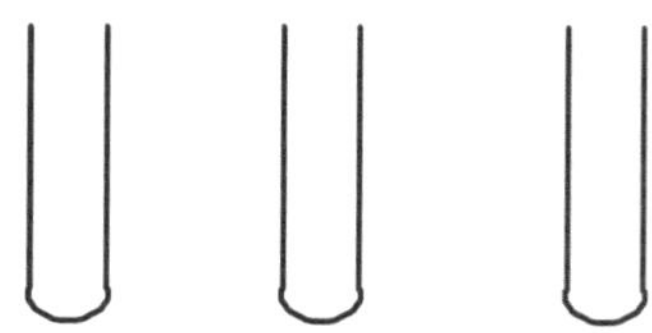

	T	S	B
1. Serum sample	0.1 ml	-	-
2. Protein standard	-	0.1 ml	-
3. Distilled water	-	-	0.1 ml
4. Biuret reagent	5.0 ml	5.0 ml	5.0 ml

5. Mix well and keep the tubes at 37°C for 10 minutes during which a purple colour will develop.
6. Cool and read the optical density at 540 nm of test and standard against the blank.

Calculation

$$\text{Concentration of total protein (g/dl)} = \frac{\text{O.D. of Test}}{\text{O.D. of Std.}} \quad \text{Conc. of Std.}$$

Result : Protein concentration of the given plasma / serum is ___________g / dl.

Interpretation

Albumin

Principle: Albumin in serum binds with Bromocresol green dye at specific pH. At a pH of 2-4; Bromocresol green forms green colored complex with albumin. The absorbance of which is measured at 600 nm.

Reagent

1. *Standard Albumin :* 6 gm/ 100ml
2. *Bromocresol green :* dissolve 8.85 g of succinic acid108 mg sodium salt of BCG and 100 mg of Sodium acid in about 250 m of water add 4 ml of 30% Brig -35. Adjust pH to 4.2 0 with 1 mol/l NaOH and make up to 1 litre with water.

Procedure

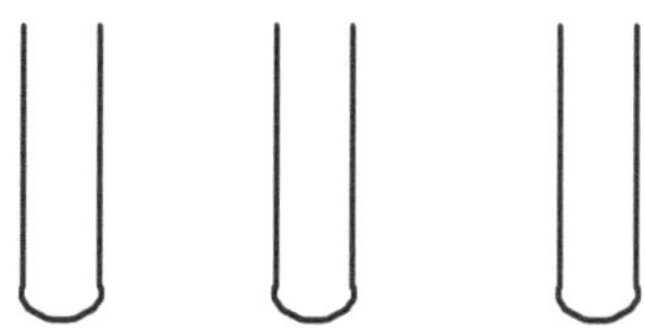

	T	S	B
1. Serum sample	0.03 ml	-	-
2. Albumin standard-	0.03 ml	-	
3. Distilled water	-	-	0.03 ml
4. Bromocresol green	4.5 ml	4.5 ml	4.5 ml

5. Mix well, and allow tubes to stand for 1 min. at room temperature.
6. Measure O.D. of standard and test with red filter at 500 nm against blank using spectrophotometer.

Calculation

$$\text{Serum albumin (g/dl)} = \frac{\text{OD of test}}{\text{OD of standard}} \text{ X Conc. Of albumin}$$

Result : Albumin concentration of the given plasma / serum is ___________g / dl.

Interpretation

Globulin

Serum globulin (g/dl) = Conc. of total protein - Conc. of albumin

A: G ratio =

Interpretation

Questions

1. Estimate the total protein, albumin and globulin in given samples.
2. Write the normal values of serum/plasma total protein, albumin, globulin and A/G ratio in different livestock.
3. Write the cause of hypoproteinemia and hyperproteinemia in cattle.
4. Write the name of conditions in which increased and decreased albumin level in serum of domestic animals.

Answer Sheet

Exercise 11

Collection, Preservation and Dispatch of Materials for the Estimation of Microminerals (Copper, Manganese, Zinc and Iron in Serum, Fodder, Concentrate Mixture and Soil) and Enzymes Like SGOT, SGPT etc.

Trace minerals have long been identified as essential components in the diets of domestic livestock species. Trace minerals exist in cells and tissues of the animal body in a variety of chemical combinations, and in characteristic concentrations, depending on the trace mineral consumed and the tissue in which it is metabolized. Concentrations of trace minerals must be maintained within narrow limits if the functional and structural integrity of the tissue is to be maintained and the growth, health, and productivity of the animal are to remain unimpaired. Minerals are as vital to cattle as grass, water or air. They play a part in essentially every aspect of growth and performance, such as reproduction, bone structure, muscle development, milk production, digestion, and metabolism, therefore, receiving greater attention for monitoring metabolic status for early diagnosis of deficiency disorders. Further, evaluation of their status in soil, plants and in animals blood is of utmost importance for sustainable development of dairy industry.

Estimation of some enzymes indicates the status of liver, kidney and muscular damage if any. These enzymes are involved in cellular metabolism of hepatocyte. Normally their concentration is extremely low in plasma but it increases many times when these hepatocytes are damaged. These enzymes are not completely specific for the liver but abnormal value gives idea about the nature and extent of the disease.

1. *Digestion of serum samples* : Two ml of serum is taken in a 150 ml conical flask and 5 ml concentrate nitric acid is added, keep at hot plate for about 30 min., cool, add 5 ml triple acid (nitric acid, perchloric acid and sulfuric acid in ratio of 10:4:1, v/v) and again place on hot plate till the contents are reduced to about 1 ml. then, after cooling volume is mad upto 10 ml with triple glass distilled water.

2. *Processing of the samples of fodder and concentrate mixtures*: the samples of fodder and concentrate mixtures fed to animals are dried first in the air and then in oven, crushed with wooden roller and kept in labeled polythene bags for future use.

3. *Digestion of samples of fodder and concentrate mixtures* : One gram of processed sample is taken in a 150 ml conical flask and 10 ml of HNO_3 is added, keep on hot plate till brown fumes subside, cool, and add 10 ml of triple acid consisting of nitric acid, perchloric acid and sulfuric acid in the ratio of 10:4:1, (v/v) and again keep at hot plate till

the contents are reduced to about 1 ml and white vapours are visible and volume is made upto 50 ml with triple glass distilled water after it is cooled properly.

4. Collection and processing of soil samples : The soil samples are collected from field where fodder fed to the animals are grown.

   1. The soil sample is collected from five spots (four corner and one central) and must be dug upto 15 cm depth in a 'V' shape taking care that all layers are included.
   2. Keep the soil on a clean cloth or gummy bag and mix well.
   3. Remove ant stones and roots and twigs of plants if seen in the soil.
   4. If the soil is wet, it should be dried it in shade.
   5. Keep the soil at one place and divide it into 4 parts i.e. A, B, C and D.
   6. Remove the parts of A and C.
   7. Mix the parts of A and C.
   8. Divide the mixture of A and C into again 4 parts i.e. into E, F, G and H.
   9. Separate E and F and mix them.
   10. Then repeat the same process once again.
   11. One should get ½ to 1 kg of soil finally.
   12. Dry the soil in the shade and fill in cloth bags with properly labeled for future use.

5. *Estimation of microminerals in serum, fodder, mineral mixure and soil :* The microminerals (Cu, Fe, Mn and Zn) are estimated by Atomic Absorption Spectrophotometer (AAS) by using different filters and wave length.

Estimation of SGOT and SGPT enzymes

Colorimetric Method

Principle : The reaction is allowed to take place by adding ketoglutaric acid and aspartic acid for AST and ketoglutaric acid and alanine for ALT. The reaction is stopped by dinitrophenyl hydrazine (DNPH) reagent. DNPH reacts with pyruvate to form a brown coloured complex in alkaline medium which is measured colorimetrically(DNPH can react with all oxoacids. It gives more colour with pyruvate, oxaloacetate and 2-oxoglutarate being 1, 0.55, 0,33 respectively. Because of the high blink value, the reaction is carried out at the suboptimal concentration of oxoglutarate).

Reagents

1. *Buffer substrate*: Phosphate buffer (100 nmol/L). Dissolve 15 gm K_2HPO_4, 2 gm KH_2PO_4 and 300 mg 2-oxoglutaric acid in 800 ml water. Adjust the pH to 7.4 with sodium hydroxide solution.

   For AST - add 13,2 gm aspartic acid.

   For ALT - add 17.8 gm D alanine and make the volume to 1 litre.

2. *DNPH reagent (1 nmol/L):* 200 mg dinitrophenyl hydrazine in 1 mol/L HCL.

3. *Sodium hydroxide solution (0.4 M) :* Dissolve 1.6 g sodium hydroxide in distilled water to make the final volume 100 ml.

4. *Pyruvate solution (2nmol/L):* Dissolve 0.176 g pyruvate in distilled water to make the final volume 1000 ml.

Protocol

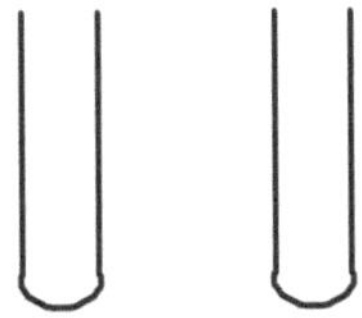

	T	B
Buffer substrate	1	1
Incubate at 37° C x 3 min. Serum	 0.2 -	 -
Incubate at 37° C x 3 min. for ALT and 60 min. for AST		
DNPH reagent	1	1
Serum	-	0.2
Remove from the water bath and keep at room temperature for 20 min.		
NAOH	10	10
Mix and keep for 5 min. read at 500-520 nm.		

A standard curve using various concentration (0.1 - 0.4 μmol of pyruvate) from pyruvate standard (reagent 4) can be prepared. The total volume of pyruvate solution should be 1.2 ml and the reaction is to be carried out as described in the protocol. The absorbance of the blank/control has to be subtracted from the test to get the actual absorbance. Transminase activity can be calculated from the calibration curve (absorbance is plotted against transaminase activity). A standard curve can also be prepared using control serum with known activity for AST and ALT.

Observations

Interpretation

Questions

1. Collect, process and estimate the trace minerals from the given animals.
2. Write the values of trace minerals in common fodders of Jammu region.

Answer Sheet

....

....

....

....

....

....

Exercise 12

Establishment of Relationship between Soil, Plants and Animals

The concentration of essential elements must be maintained within quite narrow limits if the growth, health and productivity of the animal are to be maintained. Soil-plant-animal relationship is based on micro-mineral profile in animal blood, plant (fodder) and the soil is of paramount importance to identify dietary requirements of animals maintained under different husbandry practices of various agro-climatic zones. The soil occupies a strategic position in the chain of nutrition flow to plant, animal and eventually to man. The soil is the principal source of trace elements entering the food chain. The influence of the chemical composition of soil on the trace element contents of pant is well known.

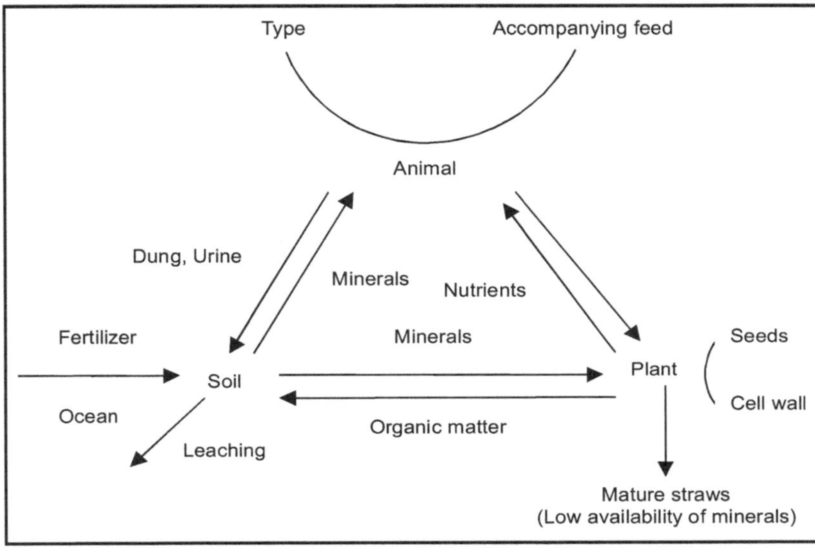

Source: Adopted from practical manual (VCM-512), Veterinary College, Chennai.

Soil-plant and animal interrelationship

The plants derive their minerals from soil and the animals from the plants/feed they consume. Because of soil-plant-animals relationship deficiencies observed in soil are generally reflected in animal's inspite of the regular supplementation of the animal diet with mineral mixture containing the trace minerals. It is worth mentioning that the supplementation of animal diets with mineral mixture as per ISI specifications may not necessarily fulfill the trace element requirement of herds maintained under different geographical and agro-climatic conditions. Therefore, one standard recommendation for element supplementation may not be suitable to delineate trace element deficiencies from entire country. Therefore, this is the high time to prepare zonal maps for trace element status of soil so as to enrich the soil vis-à-vis animal diet for specific trace element (s) for sustainable animal husbandry in India through effective herd health programme.

Identify the soil-plant-animal relationship on the basis of observations recorded in exercise no.11.

Observations

Interpretation

Questions

1. Write copper, iron, manganese and zinc values in different types of soil in our region.
2. What is the relationship between copper, molybdenum and sulphur in soil, fodder and plasma of animals of same region?

Answer Sheet

....

....

....

....

....

....

Exercise 13

Test Therapy and Examination of Blood, Urine and Milk for Ketone Bodies

Increased ketone bodies level in blood, known as ketonemia and condition is ketosis. The disease respond readily to treatment with glucogenic substances which can be one of the test therapy to differentiate this condition from milk fever and hypomagnesemia. The efficacy of this therapy can be estimates through estimation.

Collection of blood samples

Collection of blood sample is already discussed in exercise no. 4.

Collection of urine samples

Urine sample can be collected in a suitable vessel during spontaneous or induced urination, or by catheterizing the animal. In cows, gently rubbing the perineum a short distance from the vulva will often stimulate urination; laying down on straw bedding in the box or stall has the same effect in the horse; in male sheep diuresis is induced by occluding the nostrils for a few seconds. Pouring cold water over head and back may some time induce urination.

Collection of milk samples

Milk sample should be collected in the screw caped vial after proper cleaning of teats with 70% alcohol and avoid extraneous contamination. Firs few strips should be discarded.

Determination of ketone bodies

Ketone bodies are normal end products of lipid metabolism formed as a result of breakdown of fatty acids and accumulation of acetyl co-enzymes. Ketone bodies are acetone, acetoacetic acid and b-hydroxybutyric acid, which are present in different concentrations. When their blood levels raised above threshold level then comes out in the urine and milk. Urine samples are more sensitive for ketone bodies than milk.

1. Acetone in urine/milk/blood

(I) Ross test

The principal of this test is that sodium nitroprusside is decomposed to sodium ferrocyanide, sodium nitrite and ferric hydroxide in an alkaline solution. These oxidizing agents form complex having purple colour in the presence of diacetic acid and acetone.

Procedure

Prepare a reagent powder by mixing 1 part sodium nitroprusside and 100 parts ammonium sulfate.

Take 0.5 gm of powdered reagent in a dry test tube

↓

Add 5 ml of sample and agitate

↓

Add 1-2 ml concentrated ammonium hydroxide solution

↓

Note the color and graded on the basis of color as-

Trace	:	Very slight purple color
+	:	Slight purple color
++	:	Moderate purple color
+++	:	Dark purple color
++++	:	Dark purple to black color

(II) Rothera's test

Several modifications of the test exist for field use. A modified method using a mixed powdered reagent consisting of 100 gm ammonium sulfate, 50 gm sodium carbonate and 3 gm sodium nitroprusside. The powder is kept away from the moisture.

Take 1-2 gm of reagent powder in a dry test tube

↓

Sample is run down from the side of the tube

↓

Forms a layer on the top of the reagent wait for few minutes for development of violet colored ring without disturbing

↓

Violet colored ring indicates positive reaction

2. Acetoacetic acid in urine/milk/blood

Take 10 ml sample in test tube

↓

Add 5 drops of 30% acetic acid

↓

Add 5 drops of Lugol's iodine

↓

Add 3 ml of chloroform

↓

Mix them properly and allow to stand for change of colour

↓

If solution remains colorless, indicate positive test

↓

while in negative test it may have a reddish violet colour

3. β-hydroxybutyric acid in urine/milk/blood

Take 20 ml sample in a small beaker
↓
Add 20 ml distilled water
↓
Add few drops of acetic acid
↓
Boil the contents over flame till it remains 10 ml
↓
Add 1 ml hydrogen peroxide and warm it for 1 min, and then cool it
↓
Overlay strong ammonia water and allow to stand for 3-4 hours
↓
Purple colour ring is formed in positive test

Observations

Interpretation

Questions

1. Define the test therapy and explain with examples.
2. Write the normal values of ketone bodies in different body fluids of the domestic animals.

Answer Sheet

Exercise 14

Enlisting of Vitamins and Minerals Rich Diets and Feeding Schedule During Different Stages of Life and Diseased Animals

The daily nutrient requirements of animals varies for various stages of life i.e. maintenance ration, growing, working, pregnant, lactating, dry and diseased animals ration. Maintenance ration contains the vitamins and mineral only for life without any other production, while during pregnancy and lactation their requirements changed drastically from the maintenance ration. If not supply the standard amount of vitamins and minerals during these stages may disturb the metabolism and ultimately cause the production or metabolic disease. Therefore, the proper and sufficient (as per standard requirements) supplementation of vitamins and minerals can help in the prevention and control of production diseases in livestock.

General guidelines for feeding dairy animals under Indian conditions (ICAR, 1998).

Stage of life	Composition of ration
Maintenance (400 kg live weight)	6 kg straw + 1.5 kg concentrates.
Pregnancy (400 kg live weight + last 2 month of pregnancy)	6 kg straw + 1.5 kg concentrates + 1.5 kg extra concentrate for pregnancy allowances.
Lactation	6 kg straw + 1.5 kg concentrates + 1 kg concentrate for every 2.5 kg of milk produced.

Concentrate mixture can be home made or ready made cattle feed and it should generally have 30% oil cakes, 30% cereal grains, 20% cereal byproducts and 20% gram husk. In general, roughages constitute 2/3 of total dry matter intake and concentrates 1/3 of total intake.

Daily nutrient requirements of growing dairy cattle & bulls (NRC, 1989).

	Minerals (g)		Vitamins (x 1000 IU)	
	Ca	P	A	D
I. Calves fed only milk or milk replacer				
45	8	5	1.94	0.30
II. Large breed growing females				
200	21	14	8.84	1.32
300	24	18	12.72	1.98
III. Large breed growing males				
200	22	15	8.48	1.32
300	26	20	12.72	1.98
Daily nutrient requirement of lactating and pregnant cows				
I. Mature lactating cows, maintenance				
400	16	11	30	12
II. Mature dry cows maintenance plus last 2 months of gestation				
400	26	16	30	12
III. Milk production- Nutrients/kg of milk of different fat percentage.				
Fat %				
3.0	2.73	1.68	-	-
4.0	3.21	1.98	-	-

Requirements of certain minerals for ruminants

Animal type	Ca (%)	P (%)	Mg (%)	Cu (ppm)	Zn (ppm)	Mn (ppm)	Fe (ppm)
Pre-ruminant calves	0.70	6.20	0.07	10	40	40	100
Growing calves (3-12 m)	0.50	0.31	0.16	10	40	40	50
Lactating cows	0.70	0.48	0.20	10	40	40	50
Dry pregnant cows	0.39	0.24	0.16	10	40	40	50
Mature bulls	0.30	0.19	0.16	10	40	40	50
Sheep & Goat	0.50	0.27	0.15	10	40	40	50

Mineral requirements of pregnant replacement heifers

Months since conception	**1**	**2**	**3**	**4**	**5**	**6**	**7**	**8**	**9**
Ca required (g/day)	19	20	20	10	20	20	32	33	33
P required (g/day)	12	12	11	12	12	12	20	20	20
Mineral requirements of cows									
Months since calving									
Ca required (g/day)	32	36	34	30	27	24	16	16	18
P required (g/day)	22	24	23	21	19	17	13	13	16

Requirements for normal and diseased animals

Mineral	Normal dietary requirement (Orally)	In case of diseased animals (Orally)
Cobalt	0.11 mg/kg DM (both cattle and sheep)	1 mg of cobalt/day (Eg. Cobalt sulfate in sheep) In cattle the dose may be increased 10 times.
Copper	Cattle: 10 mg/kg DM Sheep: 5 mg/kg DM	Calves: Copper sulphate 4 gms. Mature cattle: 8-10 gm (weekly for 3-5 weeks). Diet should be supplemented with $CuSO_4$ at a level of 3-5% of the total mixture.
Iodine	Cattle: 0.8-1.0 mg/kg DM (for lactating and pregnant cows). 0.1–0.3 mg/kg DM (for empty cows and calves)	Salt block should contain potassium iodate @ 200 mg/kg of salt blosk which may be used as salt licks.
Iron	Cattle : 50 ppm (for all classes) Sheep: 30-50 ppm (for allclasses)	Pig: 450 ppm
Zinc	Pigs : Supplemented the feed with Zinc sulphate or carbonate @ 50 mg of Zinc/kg OR 200 gm of Zinc carbonate or sulphate may be added to each tone of feed	Pigs : 200 gm of Zinc sulphate or carbonate per kg of feed besides the parenteral injections @ 2-4 mg/kg body weight daily for 10 days.
Selenium/ Vitamin E	Dairy calves : milk replacers are to be supplemented with ? -tocopherol acetate @ 0.1 mg/kg DM of milk replacer.	Parenteral injection + ground lime stone
Calcium	Cattle : Maintenance of mature lactating cows- 17 gm/day (add 2-3 gm of Ca to the maintenance of requirements for each kg to milk produced) Maintenance & preganancy- 23 gm/day. Sheep : Maintenance- 0.3 gm/day Lactating- 0.52 gm/day.	Parenteral injection + ground lime stone
Phosphorus	Maintenance of mature + lactating cows- 13 gm/day (Add 1.7 – 2.4 gm of P to the maintenance requirements for each kg of milk production) Maintenance & pregnancy- 18 gm/day Sheep : Maintenance- 0.28 gm/day Lactating – 0.37gm/day	Mono sodium dihydrogen phosphate @ 10-20 gm to 20 liter of water may be added.
Viyamin D	Cattle : 300 IU /kg DM Sheep : 250-300 IU/kg DM Lactating : 150 IU/kg DM	- Cattle : Usually parenteral injections are given - Oral Vitamin D @ 30-45 IU/kg b. wt. - 30-45 IU/kg b.wt. daily
Vitamin A	40 IU of Vitamin A/kg of b.wt. Supplementation diet may be @ 0 to 110 IU/kg b.wt. per day depending upon the need.	440 IU/kg b. wt.

Sources of Minerals

Element	Good sources	Medium sources
Macro-minerals		
Ca	Legume fodders (10.1-14.2%), Steamed bone meal (29%), Ca carbonate (40%) and, seeds of leguminous plants, oil seeds and molasses are also good source.	Mono calcium phosphate (16.2%) Grasses (3.7-3.8%) and hay sources (23.3%)
P	Monocalcium phosphate (18-21%), sodium phosphate (21-25%).	Steamed bone meal (12.6%), Barley, corn, sorghum, oats and wheat contains 0.03-0.42%,
Mg	Magnesium oxide (54-60%), Oil seeds (3-5.8%).	Magnesium carbonate, cereal grains (1.1-1.3%).
Na	Sodium chloride	Leguminous fodder (0.8%)
K	Potassium chloride (58%), potassium sulphate (41%)	Fresh herbage (1-6%)
S	Potassium sulphate (28%), Ca sulphate (12-20%).	Oil cakes (1.64-2.50%), green fodder (0.29-0.59%) grasses (0.1-0.4%).
Micro-minerals		
Fe	1000-5000 ppm Legume fodders, cultivated green fodders, mixed local grasses, oil seed cakes, trees leaves, meat meal and top feeds.	500-1000 ppm Cereal green fodders, oil cakes and brans, tree leaves and dry fodders.
Cu	30-70 ppm Legume fodders, cultivated green fodders, tree leaves, caster cake and ground nut haulms.	15-30 ppm Local grasses, oil cakes, cereal byproducts and top feeds.
Zn	150-300 ppm Legume fodders, oil seed cakes, bran and meat meal	15-150 ppm cultivated green fodders, Cereal green fodders, top feeds, unconventional feeds like tapioca meal, coffee husk, rubber seed cake, tree leaves like glycecidia, neem, jack and banana.
Mn	100-250 ppm Wheat bran, rice bran, paddy and ragi straw and lucern fodder.	40-100 ppm Green fodders, leafy vegetation.
I	0.1-0.7 ppm Marine products, oil seed cakes, iodized salt and yeast.	-
Co	O.2-0.6 ppm Legume fodders, animal proteins and fermented products.	-
Mo	0.5-1.5 ppm Legumes, green grasses	-

Sources of Vitamins

Name of Vitamin	Source
A	Green peppers, green plants, vegetables, carrot, sweet potatoes, tomatoes, pineapples, pears, strawberries etc.
D	Cod liver oil, Raw chicken liver, raw pork liverraw calf liver, egg yolks, cabbage, spinach, corn oil, butter, cream etc.
E	Safflower oil, corn oil, soyabean oil, peanuts, oats, wheat, rice bran, carrots, bananas, butter, milk, egg, liver etc.
K	Green tea, spinach, lettuce, Brussels sprouts, cauliflower, cabbage, green beans, beef liver, cheese, butter, eggs, oat, whole corn etc.
B-complex	Wheat germ, soyabean, whole rye, whole wheat, corn meal, pork bacon, milk whey etc.
Thiamin	
Riboflavin	Wheat, green turnip, cauliflower, beets, oats, liver, veal, pork, eggs, fish, milk, carrot etc.
Niacin	Peanuts, rice brown, barley, kale, radish, bean white, beets, peppers sweet, chicken, pork, codfish, cheese, oranges etc.
Pantothenic acid	Yeast, liver, kidney, heart, egg white, dry milk, soybeans etc.
Pyridoxin	Beef liver, chicken, pork, veal, beef, lamb, eggs, rice brown, corn, cabbage, onions, milk, butter, lettuce, beats etc.
Folic acid	Wheat bread, apples, tomatoes, raw cabbage, liver, milk etc.
Choline	Barley, wheat germ, soybean, peanuts, lettuce, rice police, milk, yolk, beef brain etc.
Cyanocobalamin	Egg, cheese, liver, kidney etc.
Biotin	Soybean, rice bran, yeast, liver, egg yolk etc.
Inositol	Grains oils, citrus legumes, fruits, milk, meat etc.
Lipoic acid	Yeast, liver etc.

Exercise 15

Collection, Evaluation, Cross-matching and Transfusion of Blood in Anaemic Patients

Transfusion therapy is basically an attempt to replace blood or its components when the life is threatened. Blood transfusion plays a life saving role in general mostly to shorten the recovery time during any severe blood loss conditions arising due to accidents, major surgical interference, haemoprotozoan diseases especially in canines during anaemic conditions due to sever helminthic infestions, tick infectation, haemophilia etc.

In livestock, diversity of blood and lack of commercially available blood typing reagents, make blood group matching and typing difficult, which results in reduced importance in veterinary practice. Blood or individual blood component is to be transferred during the following conditions-

Indications

1. In intravenous haemolytic diseases like postparturient haemoglobinuria, anaplasmosis, babesiosis and theileriosis.

2. In acute drainage of blood from body due to haemorhhage or some other causes like nitrates, cyanide, warfarin poisoning etc.
3. A general supportive measure in specific diseases such as epistaxis, haemophilia, warferrin poisoning and autoimmune haemolytic diseases etc.
4. To provide specific and non-specific antibodies.
5. Moreover, blood transfusion is indicated when haemoglobin decrease ($<$7g/dl), decreased PCV ($<$20%), decreased plasma protein concentration ($<$3.5g/dl), increased heart rate, increased respiratory rate, increased capillary refill time ($>$2 seconds) and pale mucous membrane.

Decision making

If PCV is 20% immediately after hemorrhage observe for next 24-48 hours. If PCV falls below 12%, blood transfusion is indicated and if it remains stable between 12-20% then blood transfusion is not necessary. Generally in any patient having PCV $\leq$ 15% and total protein $\leq$ 3.5gm/dl, blood transfusion should be carried out.

Selection of donor

The selection of proper donor animal for collection of blood necessitates the consideration of factors such as age (adult), general body condition (good), sex, absence of disease particularly blood protozoan, so as to avoid unwanted elements in the recipient animals. Dogs over 27 kg b.wt. can donate one full unit i.e. 450ml of blood every 3 weeks without any adverse effects or need for nutritional supplementation. It has been recommended that as much as 22 ml/kg b. wt. of blood can be taken from canine donors every 10-21 days when nutritional supplementation is given. He donor should be blood typed and screened for general health and for endemic infectious diseases. Before collection of blood from donor, hematocrit should be checked. A minmum hematocrit of 40% is acceptable. If the donors hematocrit is 40%, transfusing 2 ml per kg b. wt. of whole blood will raise the recipient hematocrit by 1 %. Greyhound dogs should be preferred as blood donors because they have PCV (>60%), easily accessible venipuncture sites, a docile disposition and a low frequency of DEA-1.1, DEA-1.2 and DEA-7 antigens.

Collection and storage of blood

During collection of blood, all aseptic precaution should always be taken. Venepuncture into the jugular vein is the method of choice in large animals, using a sterile 16-18 gauze hypodermic needle attached with rubber tube is inserted into the jugular vein of the donor and blood is allowed into the collection bottle by slowly agitating it throughout collection to ensure proper mixing of blood and anticoagulant. Usually 10-15 ml of blood per kg body weight can be drawn off at a time without risk to the donor's life. The collecting plastic bottle with required quantity and type of anticoagulant should be sterilized in autoclave at 15 pounds pressure for 15-20 minutes. In past many veterinarians evacuated glass bottles for blood collection. The advantage of glass is that the vacuum allows the blood to flow quickly. However, the disadvantage is that the vacuum creates foam that disrupts the red cells, and if needle comes out of the vein, the vacuum is lost. Another disadvantage is that glass will activate some clotting factors that you want to preserve.

Anticoagulants and preservatives

Anticoagulants differ according to usage of the blood viz. either for immediate use or future use.

Sodium citrate as 3.8% solution @ 10 ml/100 ml blood is used for immediate use while the Acid Citrate Dextrose (ACD) mixture is used @ 49 ml/350 ml blood and keeps the blood fit for transfusion for 3 weeks at 4°C.

ACD composition

Trisodium citrate	-	13.0 g
Citric acid	-	4.2 g
Dextrose	-	14.2 g
Distilled water	-	1000 ml

Another anticoagulant i.e. Citrate Phosphate Dextrose (CPD) mixture may also be used @ 75 ml of CPD solution/500 ml of blood to keep it fit for transfusion for 4 weeks at 40°F.

Composition of CPD

Trisodium citrate	-	26.5 g
Citric acid	-	3.15 g
Sodium dihydrogen phosphate	-	2.22 g
Dextrose	-	25.58 g
Distilled water	-	1000 ml

Fresh blood is more desirable for general immediate use in all species however, due to non-availability of canine donor's at a particular time blood may be required to be stored. The storage of blood results in biochemical changes referred as storage lesions such as fall in glucose, pH, pO_2, HCO_3 level and rise in lactate, pCO_2 and ammonia level.

Blood groups

There are many blood groups in animals which vary from species to species. The blood groups are determined as the autosomal dominant traits and results in the presence of specific antigens on the RBC membrane. In dogs, 8 recognized blood groups are present which are labeled as Dog Erythrocyte Antigen (DEA) but 3 groups are more common or have clinical interest e.g. DEA-1.2, DEA-1.2 and DEA-7. The ideal donor dog should be negative for DEA-1.2, DEA-1.2 and DEA-7, so as to minimize the chances of sensitizing the recipient dogs. Dogs typed as DEA-4 positive and negative to all other blood group systems are considered "universal donors".

In cattle 12 blood groups have been recognized but only two (B and J) have clinical interest, while in sheep 7 blood groups but clinical significance have only B and R blood group. Horses have 8 (A, C, D, K, P, Q, T and U) blood groups but A, C, and Q have clinical interest. Special precaution should be taken not to be transfuse Aa positive and Ae positive erythrocyte into Aa negative and Ae negative mare.

Evaluation

The blood of both donor and recipient has to be evaluated for haemoglobin and PCV before transfusion. Moreover, donor' blood has to be screened for any type of haemoprotozoan and any other infections.

1. Cross matching

Cross matching of blood is must to reduce the risk of transfusion in previously sensitized patients.

2. Direct or Tridrop method

Place 3 drops of sodium citrate solution on a clean slide. Add one drop of donor blood to the first drop; one drop of recipient's blood to the second drop and one drop of both donor and recipient's blood to the third and mix thoroughly. Agglutination of third drop indicates incompatibility and the transfusion of such blood should not be carried.

Indirect or cross reaction

Collect sera and RBCs from both donor and recipient and suspend the cells in normal saline. The donor RBC are washed 3 times with 0.9% saline, and a 4% RBC suspension in saline is made from the washed cells and used for cross matching.

a) *Major match* : The major crossmatch consists of combining equal volumes (0.1 mL) of the donor RBC suspension and recipient plasma. The control tube contains recipient RBC and recipient plasma. The samples are incubated, centrifuged, and evaluated for hemolysis or agglutination. Hemolysis is evaluated by comparing the color of the supernatant in the test sample with that of the control sample. Each sample is then gently shaken until all cells in the "button" at the bottom of the tube have returned to suspension. Again, the degree of cell clumping of the test sample is compared with that of the control sample. The test is negative or compatible when the plasma is clear and the RBC are readily suspended. A positive or incompatible test can have hemolysis or hemagglutination, or both. All tests judged macroscopically to be negative for hemagglutination should be confirmed microscopically at low power. This is particularly important in horses because their RBC tend to form rouleaux. A major cross match detects antibody in the recipient against the donors red cells, where as a minor cross match detects antibodies in the donor against the recipient red cells.

b) *Minor match* : The minor crossmatch is the reverse of the major crossmatch, ie, combining equal volumes (0.1 mL) of the recipient RBC suspension and donor plasma. The minor crossmatch is important only in species with naturally occurring isoantibodies or if the donor has been previously transfused or, in horses, previously pregnant.

3. Oehlecker's Biological test

This test is carried out under field conditions where cross matching is not possible due to inadequate laboratory facilities. Inject a small amount of blood (5-10 ml) intravenously and observe for any incompatibility symptoms in recipient which is characterized by dyspnoea, increased pulse, shivering, perspiration, excitation, defecation, urination followed by weak pulse, haemoglobinurea and collapse.

Infusion of blood

The blood should be infused slowly (80–100 drops/ minute), intravenously (in jugular vein) with a sterile hypodermic needle of 20 gauze in dogs and 18 gauze in cattle and horse. Speed of transfusion depends on the condition of the animal; however, a rate of 20-30 ml/min in bovines is safely tolerated. A blood administration set with a 170mm filter is used to prevent clots and platelet aggregates from entering the recipient. Sometimes in uncooperative animals, infusion can also be carried out through intraperitoneal route, though the rate of absorption is slower compared to intravenous. The second method is contraindicated when the animal is in a state of oligaemic shock, when intravenous infusion is obligatory. It is not recommended in cases with ascites, peritonitis, abdominal distension, peritoneal adhesions or recent abdominal surgery. Before administration, stored blood should be warmed to body temperature (37°C) especially in hypothermic patients because cold blood is viscous and tends to cause vasoconstriction and also interfere with platelet functions. A total of 4.5 liters of blood usually requires an hour to administer to a cow. An infusion rate of 10-20 ml/kg/hour is recommended for the horse. Administration of the blood at too rapid rate may cause overloading of the circulation and acute heart failure. In the event of an incompatible reaction the blood flow should be stopped immediately.

In dogs, blood is administered through cephalic, recurrent tarsal or jugular vein at the rate of 8 to 10 ml/kg b. wt./hour. The first part of transfusion is to be given very slowly and is stopped immediately if urticaria develops. The dose of 10-20 ml/kg b.wt./24 hours should not exceed unless there is continuous haemorrhage. It has been found that 20ml/kg of whole blood increases the PCV by 10%. In dog, sodium citrate is the cause overloading and failure of the heart, so the blood should be administered very slowly or anticoagulant, heparin should be used. Heparin mixed blood can be safely transfused at a fast rate either IV or intraperitonially. Transfusion can also be given intrameddulary in 10 kg bones like femur, the RBCs pass very rapidly in circulation, 95% being absorbed intact within 10 min.

Quantity of blood to be transfused

The amount of blood required for transfusion varies with the size of the recipient and the volume of blood that is lost. It is necessary to replace 30-50% of the total blood lost, and in a mature animal (500 kg) 8 liters has been recommended as a guide, but the exact amount needs to be determined. The quantity of blood to be transfused will depend on the following considerations :-

- Degree of anaemia.
- In acute haemorrhages there will be a loss of blood volume and likely hypotension but with no drop in PCV for several hours, in such cases only dextran or plasma infusion may be good enough.
- In chronic anaemia the decision to transfuse blood should be based on bone marrow response and on PCV. An animal with PCV 15% and haemoglobin 5 g% and above need not betransfused.

Dose

In small animals

It is calculated on the percentage of haemoglobin present and the percentage to which it should be elevated (minimum 75% of normal level). As the animal contains about 90 ml of blood per kg of body weight, the formulae used is:

$$\text{ml of blood need to raise Hb to } 1\% = \frac{90 \text{ x body weight (kg)}}{100}$$

$$\text{ml of blood in anticoagulant} = \frac{\text{wt.(kg) of recipient x90 x PCV(desired) – PCV(recipient)}}{\text{PCV (donor) in anticoagulant)}}$$

The dose of blood is arbitrarily said to be 10 to 20 ml/kg b. wt. but this may not be true assessment as haemoglobin concentration may not be increased to the required level.

In large animals

If normal blood volume assumed to be 8% then, first calculate the amount of blood lost as under-

$$\text{Blood loss in liters} = \frac{\text{(Normal PCV - Patient PCV)}}{\text{Normal PCV}}$$

where normal PCV = 0.08 X patient weight in Kg

Once the blood loss is calculated, then-

1. Correct only 30-50% of the total blood loss.
2. Correcting ≤ 25% will not help.
3. Attaining a PCV of 25% should be goal.
4. Crude method, if PCV of donor is 40% then 2.2 ml of such whole blood/kg b. wt. will increase PCV by 1% in recipient.

Adverse reactions and its management

During transfusion the animal should be monitored for the signs of incompatibility. Anaphylactic reactions occur more commonly and are more severe with repeated transfusion. At the third transfusion almost 50% of cattle will show a moderate to severe reaction. Generally repeated transfusions between same donor and recipient produce several types of reactions which need prompt attention. The incompatibility reactions are characterized by hiccough, dyspnoea, week pulse, shivering, sweating, increased salivation, frequent maturation and defecation etc.

Transfusion of large volume of blood may cause citrate toxicity resulting in hypocalcaemia which can be treated by administering calcium borogluconate. Similarly transfusion at a too faster rate may cause acute heart failure. These reactions respond well with an early attempt and large doses of-

- Adrenalin (1:1000) @ 5-8 ml, I/M
- Corticosteroids @ 3-5 ml, I/V
- Chlorpheniramine maleate @ 5-10 ml, I/M

Questions

1. Carry out blood transfusion after conducting cross match for the given animal.
2. What is the importance of blood transfusion in aneamic animals?
3. Write the different types of plasma expanders with dose.

Answer Sheet

....

....

Exercise 16

Collection and Examination of Cerebrospinal Fluid (CSF)

Cerebrospinal fluid is found in the ventricles, cistern of brain, canal of spinal cord and in space between piamater and arachnoid. The main source of CSF is choroids plexus in the ventricles of brain. CSF is derived from the blood plasma and therefore, it has qualitatively the same composition. But the discrepancies between the ionic concentrations in cerebrospinal fluid and blood plasma indicate that the fluid is not a simple filtrate but a product of active secretary mechanism. Functionally, CSF protects and nourishes the parenchyma and maintains homeostasis. Diagnosis of diseases of CNS posses a challenge to the clinician and confirmation of tentative diagnosis based on clinical manifestations requires cytological and biochemical examination of CSF. Removal and laboratory examination of CSF are indicated whenever there is clinical evidence suggesting CNS disease.

Indications

- In the diseases of central nervous system (CNS) as a prognostic aid.
- As therapeutic measure to remove certain amount of CSF.
- For evaluation of prognosis and effect of therapy.
- To introduce opaque substances for conducting X-ray studies.

Site of collection

Animal species	Site of collection
Bovine	Postoccipital or lumbar puncture. In lateral recumbency, postoccipital method is more suitable.
Ovine	Postoccipital puncture
Porcine	Lumbosacral puncture method is the method of choice.
Equine	Postoccipital puncture
Dog	Cisterna magna or atlanto-occipital puncture. Lumber puncture is extremely difficult due to the lumbar vertebral arches and the small subarachnoid area.

Technique

1. Lumber puncture

The CSF may either be collected under local or general anesthesia by lumber puncture. When animal is standing or lying on its brisket, insert a needle in the midline between the two tubercoxae, in the hollow between the spinous process of the last lumbar vertebra and the sacrum. The needle is 120-150 mm long and 1.5-1.8 mm diameter, fitted with a beveled stylet. At the lumbar site the needle is inserted vertically through the skin, and then slowly in a ventral or cranioventral direction.

Penetration of the duramater usually makes the animal jump. At this point the stylet is removed and a 20 ml syringe attached. If application of suction to the syringe does not produce fluid, reinsert the stylet and push the needle in another 2-3 mm. if this is not successful either, place the needle under suction and start probing further in and further out. However, this increases the risk of puncturing a blood vessel, which will contaminate the CSF with blood and render it useless for most tests.

2. Postoccipital puncture

The animal is sedated and cast. Its head is bent towards the brisket to its fullest extent, with the entire head and neck adequately resieved. The puncture site is in the midline, a handbreadth behind the poll. The needle is 120-150 mm long and 1.5-1.8 mm diameter, fitted with a beveled stylet. At the *postoccipital* site the needle is inserted precisely in the midline in the direction of the occipital bone. After reaching the bone, the needle is withdrawn a little and then reinserted at a more acute angle so that the tip of the needle passes below the occiput into the foramen magnum. Penetration of the dura mater produces a pain reaction. Upon withdrawal of the stylet, it is usual for CSF from the cerebromedullary cistern (which communicates with the 4th cerebral ventricle) to drip spontaneously from the needle, whence it can be caught in a sample tube or aspirated by syringe. Emergence of a jet of fluid is evidence of increased cerebrospinal pressure.

In either case, puncture must be performed under sterile precautions after cleaning, shaving and disinfecting the site, and using a sterile needle, in order to prevent the introduction of infection into the subarachnoid space.

Storage/preservation of CSF

For the storage or preservation of CSF, the anticoagulants are used as same as the blood. Sodium fluoride is used as anticoagulant for the estimation of glucose in CSF, while for other examinations it should be collected without any preservative. However, if the delay is expected in examination, any suitable coagulant (already discussed in blood collection exercise) can be used for the preservation of CSF.

Examination

The CSF is examined for colour, turbidity, coagulation, specific gravity, cell count, microorganism and estimation of glucose, chloride, Ca, Mg, P, K and urea. In diseased animals the CSF is opaque, of high specific gravity and contains high protein and other constituents.

Physical examination

1. *Pressure* : The pressure of CSF is determined by manometer and is expressed in mmH_2O. The pressure is measured at the time of collection of CSF, after needle inserts in the duramater and stylet is removed, the manometer is fitted over the needle to measure the pressure. CSF pressure increases in space occupying lesions of the central nervous system.

2. *Colour* : The normal CSF is crystal clear and colorless and resembles distilled water. In intracranial haemorhhages it will be red tinged. Dull red or brown fluid indicates previous hemorrhage. Xanthochromia (pale orange or yellow) is due to bilirubin from degenerating RBCs. It indicates hemorrhage of at least 2-4 days and can persist for up to 40 days. It may be associated with tumors, trauma, spinal cord compression and abscesses and can have protein concentrations greater than 400 mg%. In suppurative conditions it is creamish. It will be cloudy in bacterial meningitis.

3. *Turbidity* : Normally CSF is transparent or clear. In infections like meningitis it is turbid due to the presence

of more number of cells and protein. Bacterial meningitis may be only slightly turbid to almost pure pus which may clot. Viral encephalitis, trauma, tumor, abscess may show turbidity due to large amounts of protein, fibrin and/or cells. Red turbidity may be seen due to haemorrhages and mixing of erythrocytes.

4. *Coagulation* – The CSF from normal animals does not have the tendency of coagulation. But in abnormal conditions like acute suppurative meningitis the coagulation is seen due to increased protein and fibrinogen contents owing to the damage of blood brain barrier.
5. *pH* – The pH of normal CSF is slightly alkaline (7.2 – 7.4).
6. *Specific gravity* – Specific gravity of CSF in normal animals ranges from 1.003 to 1.008, which may increase during inflammatory conditions.

Chemical examination

1. Test for protein

Among the total protein (albumin and globulin), albumin is seen normally in the CSF of healthy animal, while globulin is of pathological interest. The increased level of globulin in CSF is reported in abscess of brain and spinal cord, convulsive state, uraemia, haemorrhages and extensive non-inflammatory degeneration of brain parenchyma.

The total protein concentration of CSF is readily determined using a trichloroacetic acid-turbidimetric procedure. The CSF proteins are precipitated by trichloroacetic acid and the resultant turbidity is measure by spectrophotometer. In this technique, 0.5 ml of CSF is combined with 1.5 ml of 5% trichloroacetic acid and allowed to react at room temperature for 5 minutes. The sample is agitated and the turbidity measured against a bovine serum albumin standard at 420 nm. The normal protein content of CSF is 12-40 mg/dl.

The CSF protein levels in normal and different disease conditions of animals.

Animal species	Normal Protein level (mg/dl)	Disease condition	Protein level (mg/dl)
Bovine	<60	Listeriosis	79
		Brain tumors	19-214
		Po lioencephalomalacia	135
		Meningoencephalitis	110 -143
Equine	<70	Equine rhinopneumonitis	278
Caprine	<40	Polioencephalomalacia	52
Canine	<48	Canine distemper	45-88
		Canine cryptococcal meningo - encephalitis	501
		Canine toxoplasmosis	94

The globulin level of CSF can be determined by the following methods

a) Foam test

Take about 1 ml CSF in a test tube and shake well. The foam will appear which would disappear within few minutes in case of normal CSF. The extent of foams would be more and for longer duration in CSF having high protein content.

b) Pandy's test

Take 1 ml of pady's reagent (10 g phenol crystals/100 ml of distilled water) and add few drops (1-2) of CSF, shake well. If turbidity or foam develops, it indicates presence of globulin. Normal CSF produces only faint turbidity. It becomes turbid (cloudy) in inflammatory conditions of brains and spinal cord which may be scored as +, ++, +++ and ++++ depending upon the intensity of turbidity. The pandy's reaction is +++ in case of meningoencephalitis of bacterial or viral origin.

c) Ross-Jones

Take 1 ml of saturated solution of ammonium sulfate in a test tube. Add 1 ml CSF along the walls of test tube slowly and the test tube is allowed to stand for 10-15 minutes. If white to grayish ring is formed at the junction of two fluids indicates presence of globulin.

d) Nonne-applet test

Take 1 ml saturated solution of ammonium suphate in a test tube and add 1 ml CSF. Mix the contents thoroughly and keep on stand for 5 min. If the protein is present in excess, then mixture becomes turbid with a cloudy precipitate. The None-applet reaction is usually ++ in viral encephalomyelitis while in bacterial encephalitis it is +++ reaction.

e) Sulfosalisylic acid test

Take 1 ml CSF in a test tube and add 3 ml of 3% sulfosalisylic acid and mix them properly. Keep on stand for 5 - 10 min. In case of high protein content the turbidity will appear which should be graded as +, ++, +++ and ++++.

2. Test for Glucose

The technique for detection of glucose in CSF is the same as that utilized for determination of glucose in blood (in exercise no.5). The concentration of glucose in CSF is approximately 60 to 70% of the total blood glucose level. In normal animals, glucose CSF values range from 40 to 80 mg/dl. The concentration of glucose in CSF is dependent upon : (1) the blood glucose level, (2) the selective permeability of the blood-cerebrospinal fluid barrier, and (3) the presence or absence of glycolytic microorganisms i.e. pyogenic organisms. As the CSF glucose level is directly related to that of serum, a serum sample should be collected at the same time as CSF and submitted for glucose analysis.

Decreased CSF glucose level (hypoglycorrhachia) is seen in hypoglycemia and in acute pyogenic infection is chiefly the result of the glycolytic activity of the pyogenic organisms.

Increased CSF glucose concentration (hyperglycorrhachia) is seen in diabetes mellitus, brain tumor, encephalitis, spinal cord compression and brain abscess.

a) Chloride

The chloride level in normal CSF is higher than the blood chloride levels. The technique for detection of glucose in CSF is the same as that utilized for determination of glucose in blood. The chloride levels of CSF is decreased in meningitis, protected vomiting and in advance cases of pneumonia. The chloride level in CSF is inversely related with protein content of CSF.

b) Other chemical examinations

Occasionally, non-protein nitrogen determination may be performed in the CSF. However, their relative concentration will differ from that found in blood. In cases of uraemia, the urea nitrogen level in CSF will increase at about the same rate that it does in blood.

Cholesterol concentration increases in haemorrhages on central nervous system, tumor, meningitis and brain abscess. The normal level of cholesterol in the CSF of domestic animals varies from none to minute traces.

Enzyme determinations have not been extensively studied. Measurement of creatinine phosphokinase (CK) activity may be of value. Plasma CK does not normally crosses the blood-brain barrier. Increased CSF creatine kinase activity has been reported in a wide variety of neurologic disorders. Elevated CSF CK levels in dogs (normal values = 3 IU/L) appears to be a nonspecific but sensitive index of CNS disease. When there is an increase in CSF-CK activity, there would be poor response to therapy with progression of the disease and death. SGOT (AST) is found to be elevated in canine distemper, purulent meningitis, or damage to brain tissue. SGPT (ALT) is found to be elevated in canine distemper.

Normal parameters of CSF in domestic animals

S. No.	Parameter	Cattle	Sheep	Goat	Horse	Pig	Dog
1.	Pressure (mmH_2O)	200	270	-	400	145	170
2.	Specific gravity	1.005-	-	-	1.004-	-	1.003-
3.	Viscosity	1.008	-	-	1.008	-	1.010
4.	Protein (mg/dl)	1.01-1.02	29-42	12.0	1.0-1.05	24-29	-
5.	Albumin (mg/dl)	16-33	-	-	29-72	17-24	11-55
6.	Globulin	-			23-68		-
	a) Nonne-applet		-ve	-ve		-ve	
	b) Pandy's	-ve	-ve	-	+	-ve	Traces
	c) Ross-Jones	-ve	-ve	-	+	-ve	Traces
7.	pH	-ve	7.35	-	+	-	-ve
8.	Glucose (mg/dl)	7.22-7.26	52-85	70	7.13-7.36	48-87	7.42
9.	Calcium (mg/dl)	35-70	5.77	4.6	75.2	-	74
10	Chloride (mg/dl)	5.1-6.3	450-521	460	5.55-6.98	-	6.56
11.	Magnesium (mg/dl)	390-435	2.86	2.28	414-475	-	485
12.	Phosphorus (mg/dl)	2.17	-	-	1.98	-	3.09
13.	Potassium (mg/dl)	1.6-1.9	-	11.6	1.44	-	-
14.	NaCl (mg/dl)	11.2-13.8	750-868	766	12.66	-	11.6
15.	Urea (mg/dl)	650-725	-	-	690-792	-	808
16.	Urea nitrogen	9.2	-	-	3.28	-	10.7
	(mg/dl)	4.4			1.68		5.1
17.	Cells (per mm^3)	0-10	0-15	1-11	4-23	1-20	0-25

Microscopic examination

The total and differential leukocyte counts are mostly preferred in CSF examination. The cell counts of CSF must be made within an hour of its collection. Cells have a tendency to degenerate rapidly because CSF is relatively protein deficient. Alternatively, equal volumes of 95% ethanol may be added to a part of the collected CSF to preserve cells. If chemical examinations are needed, CSF without alcohol should be retained. Normally CSF contains mononuclear histocytes, endothelial cells and small number of lymphocytes.

Draw WBC diluting fluid upto mark 1 in WBC pipettet and draw CSF upto mark 11 and mix thoroughly. Discard few initial drops and fill the chamber as in case of blood cell counts. Leave the chamber for 2-5 minutes and count the cells in entire ruled area multiply by 1.22 to obtain the total cells/ml of the CSF. The differential fits are made by making the smear from CSF. If the total cell count is less a 500/ml; then prepare smear from sediment of centrifuged CSF for initial cell counts. The smear is fixed and stained with Giemsa as in case of blood smears.

Normal CSF is almost cell free, having <5 nucleated cells/ml of domestic animals, which may increase to 400 cells/ml in non-purulent encephalomyelitis. Lymphocytes are mainly (70%) in the CSF. Increased number of leukocytes is known as pleocytosis, noticed in encephalitis, meningitis, abscesses of brain and spinal cord. Increased number of neutrophils is observed in pyogenic bacterial infections, abscess, bacterial encephalitis, meningitis and haemorhhages. Increased lymphocytes is seen in viral infections, chronic diseases of brain and spinal cord, toxic conditions and in uraemia. An increase in eosinophils has been reported in crptococcosis. In protozoal infections, macrophages predominate although there is also an increase in neutrophils. Continuous increase in number of neutrophils may a sign of progressive lesions which may be considered as unfavourable prognosis. If the cell patterns changes and rise in lymphocyte count is observed then it can be considered as a favourable sign of prognosis.

Observations

Interpretation

Question

1. Collect and evaluate the CSF from the given animal.

Answer Sheet

....

....

....

....

....

....

....

Exercise 17

Collection and Examination of Bone Marrow and Lymph Node Biopsy

Bone marrow biopsy

Indications

- In blood abnormalities in which it is impossible to confirm a diagnosis by means of peripheral blood examination.
- In conditions like leucopenia, non-regenerative anaemia and thrombocytopenia.
- As a confirmatory diagnosis of leukaemia and differentiating it from leukemoid reactions.

Material required

- Rubber gloves
- Anesthetic (Xylocain)
- Scalpel
- Skin disinfectant (70% alcohol)

- Syringe (12 ml) and biopsy needles (13-18 gauge, 1½-3.5 inch)

Selection of needle for aspiration biopsy of bone marrow is based on biopsy site and its depth from skin and density of bone.

Site of collection

Cattle

Bone marrow can be collected from sternum which is an easy site in young animals. In order cattle 'rib' is the appropriate site. Usually $11^{th}/12^{th}$ and about 3-4 inches below costo-vertebral joint.

Horse

Either sternum or ribs

Sheep and Goat

Sternum

Collected material may be immediately made into smear. A squash preparation is made of tissue fragments by placing a second slide firmly down on top of the particle and very carefully drawing two slides apart.

Dog

Most appropriate site is anterodorsal aspect of iliac crest. Depending upon the mental state of the animal, tranquilisers may be used. The iliac crest is outlined and the surface is prepared for aseptic surgery. Dogs can be kept in standing position or may be placed in its side by legs extending in a sitting position with legs held under the abdomen. A sterile 16 gauze needle is placed through the skin and muscle over the iliac crest. When the needle reaches medullary cavity, with the help of glass syringe a small amount of marrow fluid (0.2 to

0.5 ml) has to be collected and smears may be prepared immediately. Another site of collection is from the femur (Trochanter major).

Staining

Usually a polychrome stain such as Wright or Giemsa stain is used for staining of bone marrow smears and should be exposed to stain for longer periods than peripheral blood smears.

Examination of smear

Count 200 to 500 nucleated cells and identify red cell (erythroid) and white cell (myeloid) precursors. Determine myeloid : erythroid (M:E) ratio by dividing the number of nucleated RBCs into the sum of all cells belonging to the granulocytic series. Include different areas of the bone marrow in the cell count.

The M:E ratio is one of the important determination to be considered in evaluating bone marrow examination. M:E ratio in healthy animals most commonly range from 0.75 to 3.0. ***Increased M:E ratio*** occur in inflammatory leukocytosis, leukemoid reaction, granulocytic leukemia, lymphosarcoma and erythroid hypoplasia e.g. pure red cell aplasia, anaemia due to chronic diseases, endocrine hypofunction (thyroid, adrenal and pituitary) and infectious diseases. ***Decreased M:E ratio*** occur in myeloid hypoplasia (drug induced, immune mediated, *E. canis* infection), erythroleukemia, absolute polycythemia and regenerative anaemia.

$$\text{ME ratio} = \frac{\text{Myeloid cells of bone marrow}}{\text{Nucleated erythroid cells of the marrow}}$$

Limitations

- Many a times in most of animals it is difficult to procure the sample.

- A sample of marrow not contaminated with peripheral blood becomes difficult to collect.
- Accurate interpretation of bone marrow examination is dependent upon the ability of the individual examining the smear to different various cell types.

Lymph node biopsy

Indications

- Lymphocytic leukaemia.
- Adreno cortical insufficiency.
- In diagnosis of hyperthyroidism.
- In haemoprotozoal infections like theileriosis.

Technique

Lymph node biopsy is obtained by needle puncture method. Select a superficial lymph node, following all aseptic precautions, inject a 16 gauze needle with stilet. With the help of glass syringe aspirate few drops (about 0.5 ml) of the fluid. Some times if no fluid is coming out, inject 0.5 - 1.0 ml of normal saline and then aspirate to get sufficient fluid. The biopsy can also be obtained by puncturing the lymph node with a suitable biopsy trocar or by portioned resection or even complete removal of the lymph node after exposure through the incision.

Prepare a smear for cytological examination from aspirated fluid or directly from the freshly cut surface immediately after collection of the gland. Stain and examine the smear under microscope. Impression smear of lymph node biopsy material are prepared and examined for the confirmatory diagnosis of theileriosis. For histological examination a piece of tissue, atleast 5 - 10 mm diameter, should be packed in formaldehyde.

Smear examination

Stained smear should be examined under the microscope. Lymphocytosis is observed in lymphocytic leukaemia, post vaccination period, chronic infection and adreno-cortical infection. Lymphopenia is noticed in viral diseases, post therapy of adreno-cortical hormones and in response to stress conditions. Based on the type of cell in smear following conclusions can be drawn-

S.No.	Findings	Interpretation
1.	Lymph node enlarged with normal cell population.	Hyperplastic lymphnode
2.	Lymphnode enlarged with increase in plasma cells, lymphoblasts, macrophages with hemosiderin and debris.	Reactive lymph node
3.	Large number of non-lymphoid leukocytes present.	Lymphadenitis
4.	Nn-lymphoid cells with malignant cells.	Metastatic neoplasia
5.	Major cells are lymphoblasts	Lymphoid neoplasia

Observations

Bone marrow biopsy ....

Lymph node biopsy ....

Interpretation

Bone marrow biopsy ....

Lymph node biopsy ....

Questions

1. Collect and evaluate the bone marrow from given animal.
2. Collect and evaluate the lymph node from given animal.
3. Pictorially depict the superficial lymph nodes in ruminants, equines and canines.
4. Write composition of lymph. How it differs from blood?
5. Write the normal value of M:E ration in different livestock.

Answer Sheet

Exercise 18

Collection and Dispatch of Material for Chemical Examination in Veterolegal Cases

Samples for toxicological analysis are usually taken during post-mortem examination. In suspected cases of poisoning the following specimens should be sent for chemical analysis.

Suspected poison	Required material in order of importance
1. Alkaloids	i) Liver, ii) Urine, iii) Brain
2. Arsenic (acute)	i) Liver, ii) Kidneys, iii) Stomach contents
3. Arsenic (chronic)	i) Hair, ii) Liver, iii) Urine.
4. Copper	i) Liver.
5. Cyanide	i) Stomach contents, ii) Liver, iii) Oxalate blood.
6. Insecticides (chlorinated)	i) Fat, ii) Liver, iii) Stomach contents.
7. Insecticides	i) Oxalated blood, ii) Whole blood, (Organophosphorous) iii) Stomach contents.

8. Lead (acute)	i) Kidneys, ii) Liver, iii) Urine.
9. Lead (chronic)	i) Hair, ii) Liver, iii) Kidneys, iv) Urine.
10. Mercury	i) Liver, ii) Kidneys, iii) Stomach contents.
11. Nitrate and Nitrite	i) Stomach contents, ii) Whole blood.
12. Phosphorus	i) Stomach contents, ii) Liver iii) Oxalated blood
13. Phenols and Cresols	i) Liver, ii) Stomach contents, iii) Kidneys.
14. Rodenticides	i) Stomach contents, ii) Liver, iii) Urine.
15. Strychnine	i) Stomach contents, ii) Urine, iii) Liver.
16. Sodium chloride	i) Oxalated whole blood, ii) Brain, iii) Stomach contents, iv) Liver
17. Zinc	i) Liver, ii) Kidneys, iii) Feces.
18. Urea	i) Feed, ii) Whole blood, iii) Stomach contents.

Following are the minimum quantities of the specimens to be sent for toxicological examination-

Tissue/Organ		Quantity needed
1. Blood	-	30 to 50 ml
2. Brain	-	Entire
3. Fat	-	200 g
4. Hair	-	5 to 10 g
5. Intestinal contents	-	500 to 1000 g
6. Kidneys	-	One
7. Liver	-	500 to 1000 g
8. Stomach contents	-	500 to 1000 g in large animals and all available contents in small animals.
9. Urine	-	All available.

Sample for chemical analysis should be as fresh as possible and kept in a refrigerator or deep freeze. It is better not to add any preservative; packing with ice is preferred. Blood should not be frozen but should be transported under refrigeration. For chemical preservation, 95% ethanol, ~ 1ml/g of sample is best. Unless the viscera and other articles are forwarded to the chemical examiner, they are to be preserved for a period of six months and are then to be destroyed after obtaining the permission from the Magistrate.

When the Veterinary Officer forwards the articles to the chemical examiner, at the same time, he should address a letter to that officer on the authorized form advising him to their dispatch. This letter should contain-

1. Animal's species, age sex, identification marks and location of lesions.
2. An impression of the seal used in closing the bottle and description of the seal.
3. A list of articles forwarded and mode of transmission (by post, rail or constable).
4. A separate necropsy report should be sent.
5. Full details of the purpose for which analysis is required.
6. The bottles should be well packed to prevent breakage or leakage during transit.
7. The bottles should be labeled and properly sealed.
8. The same seal is to be used all through and the same sealing material.
9. Note the reference number of your letter of advice to the chemical examiner on the labels of the bottles.

Question

1. Write most common poisoning which occur in animals.

Answer Sheet

....

....

....

....

....

....

....

....

Exercise 19

Treatment of Casualities and Other Emergencies in Farm Stock

Certain casualties which are encountered in clinical practice are viz. acute peritonitis, anaphylactic shock, respiratory distress, cardiac arrest, ingestion of foreign bodies, hypomagnesemic tetany, diabetic ketoacidosis, toxic mastitis and poisoning. These patients required critical care, the critical patients are those patients whose conditions are capable of changing on a minute to minute or hourly basis or patients who could rapidly deteriorate in short notice. Proper treatment of emergency disease can help in the diagnosis of specific poisoning or disease on the basis of treatment response.

Snake bite

The common presenting signs of snake bite are local pain, swelling and echymoses dark sero-sanguineous fluid may ooze from the punctured wound. Hypotension, tachycardia, pulmonary edema, respiratory distress, salivation and shock. Generally signs occur within 30-60 minutes.

Treatment

- Anti-snake venum, polyvalent i/v 10-20 ml i/v or intra arterial.
- Tetanus antitoxin.
- Broad spectrum antibiotic and NSAID.
- Fluid therapy and adrenalin if required to prevent anaphylactic shock.
- Neostigmine (Myostigmine) 20-40 mg/kg, i/m or i/v.
- Corticosteroid to prevent shock.

Anaphylactic shock

Sudden and severe dyspnoea, muscle shivering, anxiety, circulatory collapse, seizers, coma and death.

Treatment

- In severe cases, immediate administration of 1:10000 epinephrine hydrochloride (adrenaline) @ 0.5 – 1.0 ml i/v in dogs and 4 – 8 ml in cattle.
- This may be followed by intramuscular administration of corticosteroids (eg. 50 to 200 mg of prednisolone sodium hemisuccinate in daogs).
- Antihistamines may also be given intramuscularly (eg. Diphenhydramine hydrochloride @ 1 – 2 mg/kg b. wt., slow i/v.

Diabetic ketoacidosis

It is the terminal result of insulin insufficiency and possible glucagons excess. It is characterized by vomiting, dehydration, hypotension, oligosuria, severe depression, epigastric pain, a strong odour of acetone on the breath, Kussmaul's breathing, diarrhea, weight loss and coma.

Treatment

In most cases the initial plasma sodium concentration is low. Hence 0.9% isotonic saline is given intramuscularly at a speed of not more than 70 ml/kg/hour.

- If bicarbonate levels can not be measured, add 10 to 20 mEq of sodium bicarbonate per liter of fluid.
- Regular insulin may be administered @ 0.5 to 1.0 unit/kg/hour mixed with Ringer's lactate as (slow) intravenous infusion or 1/4th of the calculated dose may be given intravenously, while the remaining intramuscularly.

Check urinary glucose every hour and when the glucose levels fall below "+ +" (or a blood glucose value of 250 mg/dl) the i/v fluids should be changed to 5% dextrose solution. When the blood sugar is between 150-250 mg/dl. Ringer's lactate may be given besides regular insulin @ 0.5 units/kg b. wt. subcutaneously until the animal is stabilized. Then therapy may be begun as for an uncomplicated diabetic with an intermediate or long acting insulin preparation.

Hydrocyanic acid poisoning

Ingestion of plants which contain cyanogenetic glucosides results in hydrocyanic acid poisoning e.g. Sorghum, sugarcane, members of Brassica genus. The minmum lethal dose of hydrocyanic acid is about 2 mg/kg b. wt. for cattle and sheep when taken in the form of a glucoside.

Hydrocyanic acid poisoning is always acute and affected animals rarely survive for >1-2 hours. If a relatively indigested feed is ingested, symptoms like bright red mucous membranes, dyspnoea, anxiety, restlessness, moaning and convulsions are seen.

Treatment

- Sodium thiosulphate @ 660 mg/kg b. wt. i/v

  Or

- A combination of sodium thiosulphate (@ 660 mg/kg b. wt.) and sodium nitrite (22 mg/kg b. wt.).

  Or

- Traditional treatment for cattle is -

Sodium nitrite	-	5 g	
Sodium thiosulphate	-	15 g	I/V
Distilled water	-	200 ml	
For Sheep			
Sodium nitrite	-	1 g	
Sodium thiosulphate	-	3 g	I/V
Distilled water	-	50 ml	

Beside the above, 30 g of sodium thiosulphate should be given orally or intraruminally.

Nitrate and nitrite poisoning

Nitrates and nitrites are closely linked as causes of poisoning. Ingestion of large quantities of nitrates causes certain toxic symptoms besides giving rise to nitrites. The symptoms of nitrate poisoning include salivation, abdominal pain, diarrhea and vomiting even in ruminants, while in nitrite poisoning dyspnoea with gasping, rapid respiration is the predominant sign. Muscle tremors, weakness, staggering gait, severe cyanosis followed by blanching of the mucosae.

Treatment

@ Methylene blue @ 1-2 mg/kg b. wt., i/v as a 1% solution. If necessary, the treatment is repeated at 6-8 hours interval.

Organophosphorus poisoning

The symptoms of organophosphorus poisoning are salivation, lacrimation, dyspnoea, constriction of the pupils, muscle stiffness with staggering gait and convulsions.

Treatment

- Atropine @ 0.25 mg/kg b. wt., I/M. But in very sick animals $1/3^{rd}$ of the dose can be given i/v, very slowly as 2% solution.

  OR

- 2-pyridine aldoxime methiodide (2-PAM) @ 50-100 mg/kg b. wt., I/V.

Chlorinated hydrocarbons poisoning

The symptoms of chlorinated poisoning are complete anorexia, increased excitability and irritability followed by ataxia, muscle tremor, weakness, paralysis and terminal convulsions in severe cases.

Treatment

- Sedation with pentobarbital sodium which needs to be given repeatedly until the signs disappears.

Critical care

Critical care patients are those whose condition is liable to change from minute to minute or hourly basis or patients who could rapidly deteriorate in short notice. Veterinary intensive care can be defined as the continuous nursing care of critically ill patients using the optimum equipment available.

Essential equipments, other items for critical care unit-

- Varying sizes of endotracheal tubes.
- Aspirator bulbs or 50 ml syringes for gastric levage.
- Phonandoscope/Stethoscope
- Mechanical respirator.
- Electrocardograph with oscillograph.
- Complete radiograph facilities
- Endoscope, CT scan, EMG, EEG
- Cardiac defibrillator
- Pediatric incubator
- Urinary catheters
- Heating pads and lamps
- Forceps for removal of foreign objects
- Fully equipped Operation theater with surgical instruments, and emergency drugs.
- Bandages, blankets etc.

Essential drugs

Atropine, adrenaline, coramine, corticosteroids, NSAIDS, bronchodilators, anticonvulsants, antiemetics, antidotes for common poisons and different drugs.

Basic tests to be performed

Hb, PCV, total solids, blood glucose, BUN and urine specific gravity.

Questions

1. Write the most common causes of increased central venous pressure (CPV) in animals.
2. Write in detail about resuscitation in critical patients.

Answer Sheet

Exercise 20

Clinical Case Record

CLINICAL CASE RECORD

Case No.......... **Date..............**

Clinician (Name)

Description of animal: Species .... Breed ....

Age .... Sex ....

Weight .... Color ....

Owner's name & Address ....

History

1) Previous illness

i. Number of animals affected
ii. Whether protected against specific diseases.

2) Present illness

i) Duration
ii) Food given
iii) Symptoms noticed by owner

Clinical examination (Encircle and explain in detail below) :

Clinical examination (Encircle and explain in detail below) :

Temp. Pulse Respiration

General appearance	N	A	Thorax (Gen. appearance)	N	A
Skin	N	A	Lungs	N	A
Head (Gen. appearance)	N	A	Heart	N	A
Eyes	N	A	Other	N	A
Ears	N	A			
			Abdomen-		
Mouth	N	A	Pelvis (Gen. appearance)	N	A
Mucous membranes	N	A	Gastrointestinal tract	N	A
			Urinary tract	N	A
Teeth	N	A	Genital tract	N	A
Pharynx	N	A	Mammary gland	N	A
Tonsils	N	A	Musculoskeletal system	N	A
Nose	N	A	Limbs (specify)	N	A
Lymph nodes	N	A	Others	N	A

N = Normal, A = Abnormal

Explanation: (Explain in detail any area in which 'A' is encircled)

Laboratory Examination

Blood ....

Urine ....

Faeces ....

Milk ....

Ultrasound ....

X-Ray ....

Drug sensitivity ....

Diagnosis : Tentative ...., Final ....

Prognosis :

Treatment :

Date	Clinical observation	Medication

Fate of animal :

Sig. of Student

Sig. of Clinician

FSC
www.fsc.org
MIX
Papier | Fördert gute Waldnutzung
FSC® C083411

Zeitfracht Medien GmbH
Ferdinand-Jühlke-Straße 7
99095 Erfurt, Deutschland
produktsicherheit@kolibri360.de